Altered States

The Inside Story of Excess and Successful Recovery

Dr. Terry Neher

authorHOUSE®

AuthorHouse™
1663 Liberty Drive
Bloomington, IN 47403
www.authorhouse.com
Phone: 1-800-839-8640

First published by AuthorHouse 2/25/2011

ISBN: 978-1-4567-3375-9 (e)
ISBN: 978-1-4567-3376-6 (dj)
ISBN: 978-1-4567-3377-3 (sc)

Library of Congress Control Number: 2011902554

Printed in the United States of America

My goal for this book is to prime the pump for change.

Special Thanks To:

Albert Bieser, President and CEO NeuroGenesis, Inc. for his personal, professional, and financial efforts to provide science based recovery support for those suffering the consequences of addictions and life trauma..

Richard Andrews for his unwavering support and understanding of the need to gain better understanding of recovery needs not being addressed by "traditional" treatment services.

E. Shawn Heelan whose history of a life being lived in "**Altered States**" was the impetus for this writing and who continues to serve as evidence that even the most severely addicted persons can recover if the guidance is correct and individually constructed.

And to my wife **Shirley Neher** who never stopped encouraging these efforts.

Table of Contents

Introduction

Over the last 25 years I have presented my understanding and ideas about addictions and recovery to almost 200 audiences, including conferences, seminars, classes and workshops. After each of those I would always be approached and asked to "write a book" to include what I had been presenting so others would have better access to the information. My thought always was "writing a book is tremendous work" and my feeling was "it would just be another book put away on the "Self Help" shelves of bookstores". Now, as I near the end of my life, it has become important to me to do as I was asked.

I started to do this many years ago and at that time asked my wonderful wife Shirley how I should go about it. In her amazing way she said, without hesitation, "why don't you tell the inside story"? And so here we will have just that, "The Inside Story of Excess". Excess of all kinds, types, and shapes. Why do they happen? What is behind the irrational thinking, maladaptive behaviors, and questionable feelings that are the foundation for so much suffering in so many people.

Let me also acknowledge I am a recovering person for over 25 years now and 24 years ago I set about to figure out why what happened to me happened to me. I knew I wasn't "dumb", I had a doctors degree (DDS). I didn't believe I was a bad person, I tried to help as many as possible whenever I could. I wasn't a neglected child rejected by parents. Both my parents were kind people. My father, however, was an alcoholic (unknown to me during my formative years) as was his father. My mother had not one family member who had a problem with alcohol or even drank any alcohol, yet she became dependent drinking during times of stress. These factors contribute greatly to the susceptibilities we will discuss.

In The Beginning

My story is not unique in any way, very common if fact. We just have not done all we should have done to correctly deal with this problem in our country. Hopefully we will do so soon.

I don't know any way to adequately describe the situation without including myself as an example for many of the scenarios. My wish for you is that if you identify in any way with what you read that you will read on and take seriously the simple solutions for many of the problems. I did not say "easy solutions", I said simple. <u>Just do it</u>

"Mostly what I remember from earliest childhood is always being afraid. I always felt inadequate, unequal, inferior to my friends and peers. There was no particular reason for this, as I look back, it was just the way I felt inside. I thought I was "skinnier", less capable than others, even though my wonderful mother tried to assure me I was just like my friends. No matter what others said about me, it just did not internalize as positive.

As a result of this deep sense of inadequacy I tried to overcome my low self worth by being better in school than the others. I had to do more, accomplish more, get better grades than "they" did so I could be equal. It never worked. I got the better grades, got higher awards all through high school but it did not change the way I felt about myself. I was selected to be Executive Officer of the local high school ROTC (Reserve Officer Training Corp) and found this a path to ways of even more achievement. After high school I joined the Army and, using my ROTC experience, soon was ahead of the other recruits in accomplishments. During my Army basic training I was chosen "Soldier of the Month" and still it did not "make" me feel equal. During my active service I spent many hours "after work" honing my skills in my job, was chosen Soldier of the Month

3 more times over 2 plus years and still felt unequal, unworthy. I kept trying to do more to feel equal to no avail.

My first significant use of alcohol was when I turned 21 and could order a mixed drink at a bar. I asked the bartender "what was good" and he mixed a "seven and seven". This is a combination of Seagrams 7 liquor and seven up. I still can remember that day, see the bar and remember the experience. It was that day that I discovered that that drink changed the way I felt about myself. I don't remember how many I had, probably only 2 or 3, but my brain (I now understand) filed away the impact of that chemical on my chemistry and it never forgot it. I had a high tolerance for alcohol which I came to learn was a genetic factor from my father. I could drink several drinks and show almost no effect physiologically or behaviorally. BUT, I soon learned that between 4 and 6 drinks produced the most desired internal effects of feeling positive about myself. Of course at that time I had no idea it had anything to do with biochemistry and the chemistry of alcohol.

Upon discharge from the Army I entered college to pursue an education in the health care fields. As before I had to do better, get better grades than others to try to be equal (except when I was drinking) and this got me into professional school with minimal course work due to perfect grades in undergraduate work. Due to limited finances during this time my drinking was limited to what I could afford, but it still did for me what it had done initially, it allowed me to feel equal as long as the alcohol was on a rising level. Without my realizing it the use of alcohol was slowly increasing as the tolerance took over and it required more alcohol to do the same thing it had always done. Course work in professional school required a great deal of concentration and memorization, as well as tactical training in various skills so this also made it necessary to restrain my use of alcohol. However, when the class would "go to a party" where there was some form of alcohol I always went along and got my desired internal effect. Several of my dental school classmates have since told me that if it had not been for the help I gave them in school they would not have graduated. By overachieving in as many areas as I could I was still attempting to be equal with my classmates and graduated at the top of my class, still feeling inadequate.

Illegal drugs never became a problem for me. After all, I was a "professional" and did not do "those things", except drink daily which, I assumed, everyone else also did. (I now know that, sadly, the percentage of health care professionals using mind and mood altering drugs, including alcohol, is higher than the substance using public). Ten years into private practice I went thru a nasty divorce, lost or gave up everything I had gained, and moved to a rural area to restart my professional life. Not long after this move I married the most amazing woman I have ever known who, eventually, was largely responsible for saving my life because I was headed for destruction and death via organ failure due to the alcohol. I tried many things to somehow "fix" my life which was, by now, on a steep downhill run. I changed professions, went back to school, bought other businesses, did everything EXCEPT stop drinking, which I eventually came to understand was the problem.

In the mid 1980's I somehow made a decision to stop drinking. I still remember that morning vividly when, very hung-over, I asked God to help me "because I was sick". From that moment on I have never had a "craving" to drink. AA calls it a "spontaneous healing" and happens for some of us and not for others.

OK, I stopped drinking but I still had the original problems of inadequacy which had by now been made worse by the alcohol. What was I going to do? I could not see living the way I had, feeling as I had, and if I could not drink then what? My wife determined I could not go back to the environment I had been in, surrounded by alcohol, and so I stayed away while she liquidated our business and gave me time to stabilize. At this time a very intelligent man, Paul Nicolai who was extremely knowledgable about the effects of alcohol and alcoholism, somehow took an interest in me and he began sharing with me what he had learned about addictions. It seemed that these problems were not caused by poor moral character, or a lack of willpower, but were caused by a biochemistry deficient in certain things. When this deficiency was altered and improved by certain chemicals, like C2H5OH, ethyl alcohol, it quickly produced a dependency on alcohol to change the deficiencies to a positive balance. It was at this time that I decided to go back to school and do what was necessary to become a certified addictions counselor .

There are several books that were the best of hundreds I read at providing some answers to my questions. No one book had them all but by combining the knowledge of several writers we can gain a meaningful perspective for this purpose.

First was a book written in 1981 by Dr. James Milam and Katherine Ketchum called "Under the Influence". This book was ahead of its time and very accurate given what was understood at that time. Another was "Craving For Ecstacy" by Milkman and Sunderwirth which does a wonderful job of describing the various avenues we use to seek "normalcy". Third is a text edited by Soloman Snyder, MD., of Johns Hopkins called "Drugs and the Brain". There were many others which added bits and pieces but these, along with "The Chemical Brain" by Sidney Cohen were most helpful. Eventually the work published by Bruce Perry, MD, PhD on the chemistry and neurochemical actions in the brains of children provided the information necessary to close the gap in actual understanding of the why, what and how of the foundations for addictions and other maladaptive behaviors.

But back to the start of the process of learning and implementing.

I started eating better, taking care of myself physically, putting structure into my life, managing my life with the guidance of AA, my sponsor and my wife and very importantly, started the use of amino acids and vitamins as part of my repair plan that Paul Nicolai and I had discussed. I would take one amino acid and gauge and chart the results on my state of thinking and feeling. Then I would stop that supplement and try another and do the same charting. Eventually I came up with a series of amino acids and vitamins which, when combined, produced the overall best and most desired result. The most significant result was that I now felt positive about myself, something I had never experienced up to this point without alcohol.

I came to understand that every thought I had, every feeling I had and every behavior or action that I did was the result of brain chemistry. In a nutshell, "poor or inadequate chemistry resulted in poor or negative thoughts, feelings and actions."

Following the college studies to work as a counselor I "interned" at an outpatient treatment center, Colonial Clinic in Spokane, WA., and was assigned a caseload of early recovering men and women. I was still improving and increasing my understanding and personal use of nutritional supplements and suggested to some of my "clients" that they might want to do the same. Most did and soon became the most stable of the groups at this center, moving more quickly and more successfully into and thru the suggested processes for recovery.

One day I was reading "Professional Counselor" magazine, edited at that time by a man named Cliff Creager, and came across an advertisement for a Texas company promoting the use of amino acids and vitamins as an adjunct to the traditional addiction treatment approaches. To my amazement their formula was almost identical to what I had been using but had the added benefit of being in a single bottle. Up to that point I had to, and others did also, buy 6 or 7 bottles of various amino acids and vitamins, dole them out daily and take them at least twice a day to get maximum benefit. This was too much structure to expect early recovering persons to continue for the time needed for maximum benefit. With this product by NeuroGenesis in Houston, TX, I and my clients needed only the one bottle and could get the best benefit by taking 6 capsules a day. I tried it and it worked perfectly.

I called the company, told one of their workers (Fred Minor) of what I had been doing, what I had learned thru my experience and that of others and wanted to become associated with them. I was welcomed immediately as a source of information from not only my own experiences but from the treatment field I was involved with. I was impressed that Mr. Al Bieser, president and CEO of

NeuroGenesis, stated to me that they not only believed what I would report but would use it for more information to help others.

I started a very serious and deliberate study and documentation of brain chemistry, how it was manufactured, how it worked and what various transmitters produced our thoughts, feelings and actions. As I did this I interviewed many people with serious alcohol and other drug problems as well as persons in the community who indicated that they were under significant and long lasting stress in their lives. I documented what they described as their "feeling states", dysfunctions in their daily lives, medications they may have been prescribed and the effects, as well as any other statements they offered. All this in order to gain a more rounded understanding of brain chemistry.

When I had completed this undertaking I put together a presentation for persons at our center who were seeking help for problems with alcohol, other drugs including prescription medications, and the effects of serious (trauma) stress on their lives. I took the outline to our director, Hank Goeke, who was a long time medical professional and had an in depth understanding of human biochemistry and the interaction of medications on this biochemistry. He read the outline, looked up at me, reread the outline and said, "my Gawd man you've got it". "This explains why what has been happening has happened and gives us insight into how to correct it chemically". The success rate at the clinic began immediately to improve as clients included this information and action into their recovery plans. Another employee of Colonial Clinic, Donna Gadau, became one of the most ardent supporters of this process and does so still today.

I passed the information along to NeuroGenesis and their staff and the rest is history. I still use these products, as do my family and any friends who listen. All of us consistantly share the same great success."

CHAPTER 1

Chemical Dependencies Defined

Let's begin with a discussion related to millions of Americans, chemical dependency. In the past, chemical dependency has been characterized by such terms as "character defects," "personality traits," and sets of behaviors identified as common to chemically dependent persons.

In reality, willpower and character traits have little or nothing to do with this disease. Instead, the necessary causal factors amount to chemical deficiencies, excesses, or imbalances in the brain. These abnormal chemistries occur as a result of genetic and environmental factors beyond the control of individuals. These altered chemical states actually become the precursors or factors necessary for a person to receive positive reinforcement through the use of externally introduced chemicals.

The way we think and feel, and behaviors that result, all happen because of chemical reactions/interactions in our brains. These chemical reactions are dependent upon balanced levels of many separate chemical molecules working together with specialized brain cells called "receptors" to produces thoughts, feelings, and actions. For every thought, feeling and behavior there exists a neurochemical equivalent in the brain. As a person continues to use external chemical sources to gain thoughts, feelings, or behaviors deemed desirable, he or she becomes "chemically" dependent.

In other words, for people to become dependent on an external chemical source to produce the desired thought, feeling, or behavior, there must first exist, or be developed, a deficiency of a chemical component in their brains.

The first step toward an acceptable (for those people) lifestyle free from the need for external chemical intervention is, necessarily, abstinence from the use of these chemicals. This step, however, results in a set of dramatically uncomfortable and unacceptable thoughts, feelings, and potential behaviors as they attempt to interact in society with excessively curtailed brain-chemical capabilities.

This is the rationale for physiological stabilization as the necessary starting focus for recovery from chemical dependency. This focus is also what is lacking in many treatment experiences.

The major deterrent to chemical dependency counselors gaining a usable understanding of this process, we believe, has been the lack of practical interpretation of research findings into something we can use.

CHAPTER 2

The Disease Concept

Most in the treatment field espouse the disease concept because the American Medical Assn. has said alcoholism is a disease (AA calls it a "progressive illness"), and this makes the process "treatable". Those of us who are recovering believe ourselves to be of strong character and will, and readily accept the disease concept. Most non-recovering counselors voice the same acceptance but may, in all honesty, wonder to a degree about the claim.

In this society, a condition that meets four criteria may be termed a disease:

1. Etiology – factors that cause the condition are identifiable.
2. Symptomatology – identifiable symptoms, i.e, tolerance, blackouts, loss of control, etc. are present.
3. Morbidity – the symptoms describe a stage of the process.
4. Prognosis – in the case of chemical dependence, "guarded."

Now, **if drinking alcohol was all it takes to cause alcoholism, for example, everyone who drinks would have the disease, and not nearly everyone does.**

The etiologic factors being discussed, and the focus of this writing, are neurochemical and enzymatic. We are not discussing in depth here those liver enzyme levels and activities we know to be very important.

Approximately 50 substances naturally produced by the brain have been identified as neurotransmitters of thoughts, feelings, and actions (there are probably over 200 neurotransmitters not yet identified).. Of these, several are of special interest in chemical dependency recovery, and – very importantly – they can be identified with certain emotional states. This allows us to greatly simplify and make usable an understanding of neurochemistry.

Lets look at some of these neurochemicals and the associated thoughts, feelings, and behaviors.

Opioids – endorphins and enkephalins – are substances used by the brain to moderate pain – physical and psychological. Endorphins (endogenous morphine-like substances) seem to work to moderate physical pain. Enkephalins (met-enkephalin and leu-enkephalin) appear to have a profound effect in those neural areas associated with emotional memory. What is the most painful emotional feeling we suffer? "Low self worth!".

As a result of replicated studies, we know, for instance, that opioid levels can be influenced by genetics and/or trauma (stress). When a person's opioid availability is low, due to genetic susceptibility or unmanaged environmental trauma, that person feels incomplete, inadequate, and unworthy, due to decreased enkephalin availability. Inherited deficiencies of these chemistries are likely the cause of extreme shyness in children. They may never feel equal to their peers, regardless of reality. They always feel "second or third," never "first" or "as good as" others. When the levels of these chemistries are adequate, such as following nurturing by a parent, for example, which increases the release and utilization of endorphins/enkephalins, a child feels internally focused and calm, and has a sense of completeness. Sustained exercise releases opioids, and the person feels calm, centered, and complete ie.-euphoric.

Opiate drugs, legal or illegal, will fill these same receptor sites and produce the desired feeling of well-being. Alcohol metabolism and the eventual production of salsolinol provides the molecule that will fill enkephalin sites and increase feelings of well-being. Beer drinkers get a double dose of enkephalin replacement because, in addition to alcohol metabolism providing salsolinol, this chemical is naturally present as a result of hops fermentation in the production of beer.

Dopamine functions in areas associated with reward, pleasure, and altruism –in the frontal lobe of the brain, for instance- as well as maternal and paternal feelings associated with the limbic system. When dopamine is depleted, as in cocaine or methamphetamine use and addiction, inadequate neurotransmitter is available in these areas to produce these feelings. Consequently, addicts can not feel remorse about their actions and can not experience maternal or paternal concerns. When confronted with child neglect or abuse, for example, they typically will say they know they should care but just "can't" seem to.

Norephinephrine (NE) is produced from dopamine and is the brain's energizer/arousal neurotransmitter. When adequate norepinepherine is available, a person feels energetic, motivated, and full of "drive." If NE is lacking, a person has no energy, lacks motivation and drive, and feels "depressed".

Serotonin is the brain's emotional stabilizer. When adequate serotonin is available, a person has rational, balanced emotions. If serotonin is decreased – during premenstrual cycle, for example, or from prolonged periods of lack of direct sunlight- a person feels irritable, on the verge of tears for no reason, and can't sleep well; noises bother that individual more than usual. He or she lacks rational emotions and feels "depressed". If someone is depressed, and this depression has an aspect of irritability, then serotonin is likely low.

GABA accounts for up to 40 percent of the brain's neurotransmitters. Think of it as functioning in stress management. When adequate GABA is available, a person feels calm. When insufficient GABA levels occur, a person feels anxious for no identifiable reason (free-floating anxiety) and can experience panic attacks and eventually convulsions. GABA depletion is a major factor in delayed stress syndrome, and GABA complex depletion may contribute to various phobias, (along with serotonin depletion).

Alcohol, barbiturates (sleeping pills), and benzodiazepines (tranquilizers) all attach to GABAergic neurons and enhance the binding of GABA allowing increased chloride ions to enter the neurons, decrease firings, and producing calmness and a sense of stress reduction by reducing the fight-or –flight response.

Some enlightening studies have been published concerning enzyme and certain hormone functions. When blood samples of people involved in alcohol abuse or alcoholism were infused with the alcohol equivalent of approximately 4-6 regular drinks, regular beers or standard table wine (2.5 oz pure alcohol), certain enzymes were dramatically impacted. When control samples from individuals with no alcohol problems were tested in the same way there did not appear to be a similar impact.

One of these enzymes, monoamine oxidase (MAO), was functionally depressed, or slowed down, when contacted by the alcohol molecule in those persons drinking heavily. What can this mean? This one example significantly answers the question, "why do certain people feel energized and more alert and positive by the depressant drug alcohol"? The monoamines affected are dopamine, norepinephrine, and serotonin. MAO functions to reduce the levels of these neurotransmitters. When MAO is inhibited by alcohol, the activity level of the monoamines will increase. The result of this is increased feelings of energy (NE), increased feelings of pleasure (dopamine), and increased feelings of emotional stability (serotonin). People gaining this effect as a result of MAO inhibition feel more in control, more positive, and less depressed at four to six drinks (or the equivalent in beer or wine). This is the benefit of gulping drinks for persons susceptible to this enzyme alteration.; the quicker they get to the effective level inhibiting their MAO, the sooner they feel positive effects. MAO inhibition is also a primary factor in elevating blood pressure in susceptible individuals.

In these same studies, cortisol function was found to be lowered by the alcohol in blood samples of alcohol abusers and alcoholics. Cortisol is used by the brain to monitor threatening situations, making ready for fight or flight. When susceptible individuals lower their cortisol function with alcohol, they sense "no threat present, " no uncomfortable feelings of concern, and no reason to stop drinking. In people not experiencing this effect, their brain responds to the alcohol as a toxin and <u>increases</u> cortisol availability, making the person "uncomfortable" enough to reduce or stop drinking.

Using these few examples, then, we could say that if genetically susceptible individuals, or those who have altered their biochemistry as a result of trauma or unmanaged stress, feel more assertive, more active, less depressed, a greater sense of pleasure and calm, more stable, and more in control when they drink, and do not sense a threat from alcohol, why wouldn't they drink? **THEY DO!**

At times we hear various individuals say something like "he or she is 'too far gone' to recover. They have tried over and over and just can't seem to stay away from their "drug of choice" that has always resulted in increasing problems.

To that I say "oh yes you can"!! Let Shawn tell her story of addiction and recovery.

CHAPTER 3

My first Drink

"The first time I ever drank I was about 2 years old. My sister got into my father's liquor and fed booze into me. From what my dad now tells me, he used to give my sister and I sips of their drinks (when we were 3 and 5) as they partied with their friends and neighbors. They all thought it was amusing to watch us get buzzed.

My first conscious memory of drinking was when I was 15 and a half. Seemed like that must have been pretty important to me at the time, since the 21 year old boy that ended up raping me when I was passed out and covered in vomit, kept bringing it up to make fun of me. My girlfriend Jill and I got into her parents vodka and made ourselves vodka and Tang cocktails. Most of the evening was pretty fuzzy, but I remember feeling pretty grown up to be hanging out with Jill, her older brother who was on leave from the Navy, and one of his skuzzy friends the rapist. Her parents were out of town for the weekend. He took my virginity and left me with a badge of shame that I wore, hidden, for decades. I woke up with my pants undone and not all the way back on, blood on my thighs, and venereal warts.

The STD (sexually transmitted disease) that I contracted as a result of this encounter is what, I'm sure, caused my cervical cancer, the cancer that scarred my uterus and caused my daughter to be born so prematurely.

Some of my other memories of drinking include getting into my folks liquor cabinet and taking a little bit of all the bottles and pouring it into a container, to take with me to Skateland. I must have been in 9th grade. I'd hook up with a couple other kids who did the same thing and we would meet at the school and ride the bus together to Skate Night. We would sit in the back and sneak drinks.

What I learned about drinking right away, was that **when I drank any alcohol I felt like I fit with the crowd**. It was the only time I felt that way. I discovered that when I put alcohol into my body, I was no longer the shy geek, the ugly duckling, the girl on the fringe of the crowd, wanting so desperately to fit in but knowing I just didn't.

I never felt like I was good enough to be hanging out with whoever it was I wanted to be around – I felt "less than", inferior, like a hanger on, an imposter. I always felt like I had to buy my way in so I would provide the car, the gas money, the booze, the food, whatever. On my own I just wasn't good enough.

When I started drinking, I hated myself the next day for how I'd behaved. I wanted someone to stop me, I wanted my parents to intervene, show me they cared enough to know how confused, miserable, scared, full of anxiety I was. But when I did get confronted, either with the pile of beer caps my dad found in the car, the extra hundred miles or so I put on the car when I was just going to go "to the game", or the way I tried to sneak in hours past my curfew, it was never what I needed. It was either raging violence from my dad, who was then so sorry in the next few days that he dropped whatever consequence he had handed out, or even worse, bought me something to make himself feel better. A new car, a bike, tickets to a concert.

Then there was my mom, who taught me at a very early age that we must keep secrets. We weren't going to tell dad. She knew I "didn't mean to do" whatever it was that I did, and she knew I would be "better" next time, so we just won't tell dad. No need to make him upset. It wasn't that we were "intentionally" deceiving him, it was just that he was so busy, he loved me so much, there was no need to involve him since she "knew" it wouldn't happen again.

In my early 20's alcohol was still my "drug of choice" but I may have experimented with other "things" when with friends at a party. My memory of my life from 20 until I was almost 33 is very vague and I still only get bits and pieces even when prompted. My first real run-in with the law did not happen until I was about 25. I had been drinking "Long Island Ice Tea" (a combination of at least 4 liquors and pepsi or coke that taste like tea), several of them, got mad at my friends, got in my car and left. Very soon I was pulled over by a police officer for weaving over the center line. I remember I had on high heels and he told me to walk a line in the gravel, which I refused to do. He told me he was going to administer a "breathalyzer" which I refused, and I got belligerent. I recall several officers grabbing me and forcing me against the police car and while they were attempting to handcuff me I grabbed one of the officers between his legs and started yanking. They proceeded to forcefully restrain me and took me to jail.

I went before a judge and was "sentenced" to an "alcohol awareness class" for DUI offenders. This consisted of some lectures about the evil of drinking and I was required to meet 1 on 1 with a counselor each week for 4 weeks. After the first counseling session the counselor offered me cocaine. The next week we met at my house and used cocaine again. His behavior became very bizarre and as soon as my "required" attendance was done I got away from him.

My drinking continued to escalate and my behavior became more and more troublesome to my family. I agreed to see a psychiatrist at my parents' insistence and met with him for many sessions over the next 2 or 3 years, while continuing to drink since my problem must have been "mental" and not the alcohol. Finally the psychiatrist decided, since none of his "therapy" had fixed me, that I must be alcoholic. What a concept!

My first experience with "real" treatment was approximately 1987. Another run in of some kind with the law required an "evaluation screening" and it was determined I was "alcoholic". This center's program was 2 weeks inpatient, 3 weeks outpatient. I recall there were many classes and counseling sessions required and we were expected to "work" the first 5 steps of AA in the first 2 or 3 weeks. There was so much information and expectation that I achieved only enough to satisfy the counselor. During this time I was served divorce and custody papers while in treatment. My husband had physical custody of the kids. It was a complete uphill battle from there, as he maintained custody during a very ugly divorce. I, and others, learned quickly that the way to keep the counselors happy was to say whatever they wanted to hear. I became very resentful because, in my mind, none of the things they pushed at us seemed to apply to me and my problems. I did and said what I needed to and as a result I "graduated" with honors, told my alcohol problem was "minimal" and was pronounced "cured".

Since I had been "cured" it seemed OK to drink, as long as I was careful to not "overdrink". At the same time I was using cocaine on and off and again was stopped while driving and arrested for possession of a controlled substance. As a result of this occurrence I was sentenced to a "Women's Treatment Center". This was a very expensive program and it soon became clear that "men" were a big part of everyone's problem. There were many women in treatment who acknowledged they were "lesbian" which made me uncomfortable and I spent my "time" there isolating from the treatment population until I could be discharged. Again, I was "cured".

All of my "8 or 10 treatment" experiences had been, and continued to be, associated with legal problems. Following another arrest I was "sentenced" to an outpatient treatment program. I began to recognize that a "problem" was there and kept wondering "why can't I stop drinking?" "Why did I keep getting in trouble?" Here we went to many AA meetings as part of treatment, saw videos about using and the focus was always "just stop drinking" and you will be OK. By now everything in the treatment "program" was absolutely predictable. I had heard it all before, seen it all before. Same things over and over and I was always trying to figure out "why" it was happening" since I wanted to get sober but somehow could not see how to go about it. I was always 100% vested in what the programs said would make me "well". **I also knew that going thru what I kept going thru as "treatment" had become a waste of time.**

Shortly after discharge I was on another binge, and another arrest. I was ordered to another outpatient treatment program here and was told I "had to hit the ground running" with meetings every day, many things to accomplish. My plate was so full that the stress of it led to another relapse so I was sent to another inpatient program. Here was the same predictable routine- up early, work around the center, go to meetings, watch movies, and write a "forgiveness letter" to myself. What a joke, it seemed to me. Inundated with statistics about drinking and death, and everything in between. Graduated again and told to restrict sugar and caffeine and I would be OK.

Another relapse, another treatment center where the director told me my family was very sick, and that my husband was the "sickest" co-dependent she had ever seen. (My husband then read "co-dependent no more", attended a few al-anon meetings and announced himself cured). I, however, was a victim of circumstances and had an excellent prognosis. All of us got sick with hepatitis A. This was a Co-ed center and even though I was married, would have fraternized if there had been any available takers.

I was forced to attend another treatment center after a long run on coke that ended when two brutal people kept me hostage in a hotel in a nearby town for a couple days, beating me and then tried to kill me. I jumped thru the window to get away. I woke up in Tacoma General Hospital, not knowing who I was or where I was.

This is where I was tested for the first two days and given the diagnosis of Borderline Personality Disorder. The psychiatrist told me I would probably not live to be 40. That was such a loooooong way off, I couldn't even wrap my mind around how old that was. However, once again, I got an amazing discharge summary and was pronounced cured, again.

Sometime in the early 1990's. I went to a well known treatment center in Phoenix. I can't remember the name of the place. It was "off the wall" dysfunctional, with patients being in charge of dispensing meds, which most of the patients were taking, including methadone, pain meds, etc. I left that place and ended up staying in Phoenix and moving into an apartment complex that had a lot of people in recovery, but soon returned home to Washington.

In 1993, after another stint in jail, I went to an outpatient center in Western Washington. I had been there before but this center had a connection with the court system and didn't know my full history. I was assigned a counselor that, I now understand, was meant to be in my life. For the very first time I was "given permission" to recover at the rate I was capable of. We didn't talk about alcohol and drugs, we talked about rest, nutrition, dealing with what came up. For the first time I realized someone was really trying to support me and I didn't sense the need to lie or talk my way around things. No classes, no movies, just one on one direct support with MY problems as the focus."

CHAPTER 4

Dr. Neher's Short Story

Dr. Neher's shortened version of this very long, frustrating story:

In 1993 I was working as a counselor in an outpatient chemical dependency treatment agency in Western Washington State. Each Monday we would go over the potential intake files for new persons having made an appointment for an evaluation and possible placement in treatment. The person leading the discussion came to one file and said "I know this family and this person is never going to make it. She has been in multiple treatment centers and always goes back to her drugs and illegal actions. Her family is too enmeshed in the problems to be part of any solution". (In other words, she was a loser so why bother?) I said, "let me have the file and I'll see what I can do".

On Wednesday she came in for the assessment and we went into my office. She sat down, slumped really, and just looked at the floor. This was a 33 year old woman from a successful family and she looked like she had just come in from a bad rainstorm. Her complexion was a "nice" gray, and she appeared like what you would think an inmate in jail might look like. With good reason, actually, because she had been in jail up until 5 days previous.

I let her sit for a few minutes and then said in a very

straightforward way "you are the sickest addict I have ever seen". This jolted her a little and she sat up a little straighter, still looking at the floor. I then asked her "what are you going to do about it?" She looked at me then and said, "I don't know what to do" which is what I wanted her to say. I said, "I do know what to do". "I can tell you what to do and if you do exactly as I say you can overcome this". She began telling me that she really didn't think so because every treatment center she had been in told her was OK before she left and she seldom was able to stay clean more than a few days after leaving. Inpatient, outpatient, court ordered, family ordered, it didn't matter. She was unable to overcome this addiction to alcohol, stimulant drugs and compulsive behaviors that were ruining her life. When she needed money for drugs she would steal her parents credit cards, or charge excessively on them. As a "true arousal addict" she would put herself in very threatening situations for the "thrill" of it and several times narrowly escaped death as a result.

Again, I asked if she was willing to do just what I said, and only that, and communicate with me every day, in the office or by phone (my choice, not hers). I was very careful to not appear or sound sympathetic, and used my best "I am the boss" approach. If I had done anything else she would have agreed with me but immediately discounted anything I said. I told her all I wanted her to do for the next 3 days was eat "something" 3 times a day and stay home. She was living with her parents again at this time. No "going out" for anything. Eat, rest and call me every day.

I told the clinic that she was gong to be an "individual client" for some time and I would decide if and when she entered the standard "program". I called her probation officer and he said the same things to me – "she has never been able to make it so what is different this time?" I briefly described what we were going to do and that I would keep him updated weekly. He agreed to let her be involved.

When she came back in Friday of that week she had "cleaned up" and looked and sounded somewhat better. I outlined for her what I wanted her to do and told her not to try to remember what was discussed (because she could not remember at that point) but that I would give her, in writing, just what I wanted her to do daily. To start, I outlined a simple nutritional program, nothing outlandish but structured to begin "physiological stabilization". I then gave her a bottle of an amino acid, vitamin formulation from Neurogenesis, tailored for stimulant drug recovery. I wrote down how many to take and when and reinforced the daily eating program.

In a week she was responding well and "told" me she was going to start working out at the local health club. I said NO! I don't want you to do that yet. You can walk around the block at home and that is all. She did as I said, at least for a short time. I explained that if she was to work out heavily she would immediately crave cocaine and it would be fierce. Long story short, she did it anyway and called me in panic and said she was having intense cravings and didn't know if she could resist them or not. I told her to come to my office immediately. By doing the excessive exercise she had raised her heart rate to the same level experienced when using cocaine, or the other stimulant activities she used to do. When that happened her brain got the message she was "using" again and when she tried to stop the exercise she went into immediate "drug withdrawal". But on a positive note, she had become aware of the problems associated with heavy exercise for her and also got the message that maybe I knew what I was talking about.

For the next several weeks we stayed on this limited program and included meeting face to face 3 times a week. She rapidly stabilized and when I thought she was up to adding something to her "program" we did so. I ask her to list what she considered the three major stressors in her life, just a list, no real elaboration. Money for survival was no real issue since her folks could afford to help her and let her live with them. She didn't have a job so that wasn't' where we went. She did, however, have children who were with their father and she wanted to begin to again be part of their lives. We worked out a structure for that, discussed it with her ex-husband, and began that process. Still on her eating plan, light exercise and daily contact with me and weekly contact with probation.

Then came what I really did not want to see happen, but didn't surprise me. She met a man who she believed she could fall in love with. One problem was he was an active cocaine addict. Surprise!! She was sure, though, that she could change him. "No you can't", I told her but, like so many before her, believed if she just cared enough he would stop. He led her into relapse, and now we had double trouble. Sick relationship, relapse, probation issues, just to name a few.

She got pregnant and now, even though she was again on her recovery plan, still in the throes of a dysfunctional, cocaine dependent relationship. Eventually she came to realize that it was not going to work regardless of how many times he said he would "stop using". Now she was on her own again but with a child that was, to some degree, drug effected due to her use and the fathers use of cocaine. (Just so you know, she has taken the correct steps to help the child overcome these issues).

Now it was time to begin helping her develop life management skills so that the stress of things like paying bills, getting a job, staying out of bad relationships, etc, did not derail her again. She came over to our house in the evenings and my wife, Shirley, taught her about keeping a check book, about how to put money in savings, how to budget her money and not use credit cards you can't afford, how to itemize, on paper, your bills and what needs to be done when. (This one approach for every patient in chemical dependency treatment would dramatically improve success rates, but no one seems to want to do it.)

There was little sense in making her go thru various recovery groups except those that pertained to her issues. She could "teach" the classes on chemical dependency, family positions, etc. All the things we attempt to "teach" toxic brains with absolutely no success. But we keep doing it and charging for it.

Shawn continued her nutritional and supplement program and now, after several close "calls" had achieved 3 or 4 years of clean and sober living. She was taking care of herself and her children, was taking various classes at a community college, and working part time at her parents place of business. She and I both knew, however, that there was a real possibility that one of the prosecuting attorney's she had crossed swords with in her past may well decide to re-open her case. And so it happened and she was called into court to answer charges from the past of "possession with intent to deliver". She dealt with this forthrightly but was sentenced to a prison term of 60 months (but only served 18 months due to her good behavior and efforts). She made arrangements for her children and her mother agreed to take them until she returned. While in prison she availed herself of every opportunity to study and learn in an effort to prepare herself to once again become a functional parent and citizen. We stayed in contact during this time and I reviewed writings she did and actually communicated with one of the prison officials for help with direction for her while incarcerated. Coincidentally this prison official had attended one of my seminars in her education for her job with inmates.

When she was released she immediately contacted me and we set about writing plans for the actions she would take in developing an ongoing healthy and quality life. She considered many things to undertake, discussed them with me, looked at others and finally decided she would go to college, pursue a degree and see where it led.

Now an extremely capable manager of her life, and highly responsible for her family, she was able to incorporate several things into her development. Not only did she graduate from one of the most prestigious colleges in the State but she graduated Summa Cum Laudae. She is now one of the operating officers of the company where she works and is a source of suggestions and guidance for me and my family when we have need. I would place my life in her hands without fear at any time.

Wait a minute: this is the person who in 1993 was lost, not worth any further effort. So addicted she could not remember the previous days activity. The woman who had used drugs for years and years, heavily, anything she could get her hands on. The woman who would steal anything she could to get the drugs. She had been through "treatment" so many times she could teach the classes. Yet, here she was, successful, responsible, trustworthy, and drug free.

You say you can't make it. Oh yes you can. Just do the right things, take the right paths, make the right efforts. Yes you can, **Just Do It**.

CHAPTER 5

How did I know this would work?

In 1989 the Division of Children and Family Services, Child Protective Services, in a Central Washington city had asked me to be the chemical dependency consultant for a project they had received funding to undertake. Like most CPS offices they saw their clients, particularly mothers, process thru "treatment" time and again only to return to the use of drugs. These young mothers had already lost one child to CPS and were in danger of losing their others.

The leaders of this "program", and the persons responsible for obtaining funding for the project, were Dean Reiman and Pat Boggess. Long time CPS workers they were tired of the constant problems around drugs and relapse experienced by their clients. If "treatment" was not going to work then why continue to spend public dollars only to see them return to drug use?

I designed the program this way: We would provide "recovery services" (not "treatment" because we were not a "licensed" treatment agency) within the CPS office. We would start 12 women at a time in a "recovery group" and they would come in and meet and get acquainted with their social worker, their financial worker, and anyone else involved in the social services they were receiving. Benefit – they no longer feared these workers but came to understand they wanted to help. I traveled to this city every weekend for 2 years and on Saturdays would have the ladies come into the CPS office and we would have a one on one session to discuss the problems in their lives. On Sundays they came in and we had a discussion group about problems they faced everyday, particularly those problems associated with some aspect of drug use. Other problems discussed centered around the person they were in a relationship with, friends who used drugs all around them, disagreements they had with various people, the normal life issues we all face. (In one of these sessions three of the ladies discovered that they were all having a relationship with the same man. When the sparks diminished and I saw the disgust in their eyes I almost felt sorry for what was going to happen to him when they confronted him. I never brought it up again and they all seemed satisfied with their actions).

At this same time we asked each of the women to take an amino acid, vitamin and mineral combination provided for them at no cost by Neurogenesis, Inc. of Houston, Texas.

On Mondays they came into the CPS office and we had a local nurse talk to them about health issues, the value of cleanliness, how to care properly for their children and themselves.

On Tuesdays at the CPS office one of the financial workers talked to the group about how to budget their money, how to keep track of their bills, how to get foodstamps. Then we took them to the grocery store and showed them how to shop effectively with their foodstamps.

On Wednesdays a beautician would come in and worked with them on how to properly use makeup, do their hair various ways, and where and how to get the products they needed at the best prices.

On Thursdays the group divided up in 3's and went to each others apartments and "cleaned house". They soon learned the value of real friendships and what could be gained from working together.

On Fridays it was exercise day and they went to the local high school and one of the coaches would lead them in mild exercise and if they were unable to do the exercises they walked around the "track" as exercise.

On Saturdays it was back to me and a discussion of what was going on.

Dean Reiman and Pat Boggess would reinforce the value of this information each day as "workers" concerned for the ladies well being.

We altered the focus of these daily meetings but it was always life management issues. We would talk about the specific problems they were having and problem solve each one.

Why does this work? Because "stress – trauma" are the predictors of relapse. Deal with the problems before they become traumatic and you prevent relapse. The nutritional supplements provided by Neurogenesis made it possible for these previously "never going to make it women" to regain their neurochemical abilities to think, feel and act rationally. As their brains became increasingly capable of internalizing information they gained more and more skills in managing their lives. They left their relationships that were dysfunctional and drug infested.

Over a two year period we had over one hundred women who were "lost" not only regain their lives but become very functional and productive members of society. Some went back to school, some opened businesses, some gained meaningful relationships. All but 5 remained drug and alcohol free over the two year period. Why did this work - because we followed Mazlow's direction, applied the reality of precursor loading of correct and specific nutritional supplements, and gave them the understanding and skills necessary to deal with the problems in their lives.

The directors of the project, Dean Reiman and Pat Boggess did a terrific job of writing up the details of the project, the methods and positive results and presented this at the National meeting of Children's Services. It was rejected as "unbelievable". It seems we just do not want to learn.

These are just two of hundreds, literally thousands, of stories of those who have been willing to do what ever necessary to change their lives and were fortunate to get the correct directions.

Taking away the drugs or alcohol or dysfunctional behaviors and leaving the person with severely depleted biochemical, personal and social systems is nothing more than setting them up for failure. Look at page 64 of the Big Book of AA. On line 5 Bill W states this - "Our liquor was but a symptom. We needed to look at causes and conditions." The "causes and conditions" are those biochemical, personal, and social shortcomings we must develop solutions for and overcome. **JUST DO IT!!**

CHAPTER 6

Behavior Can Cause The Compulsion

Individuals can become addicted to compulsive, destructive behaviors due to changes in brain chemistries as a result of their behavior. Gamblers and compulsive shoppers cause a norepinephrine and dopamine rush by "betting" and "buying." This rewarding rush of energy and pleasure will temporarily "lift" depression and also substitute for feelings of inadequacy.

Starvation, as in anorexia, causes increased enkephalin levels in the brain. This functions as a survival mechanism to keep individuals calm while a food source is found. Since these people may take in no dietary source for enkephallin, they must emaciate their own muscle tissue for protein to produce enkephalin.

Bulimics cause a rush of norepinepherine and dopamine when they purge and, consequently, gain a sense of energetic and pleasurable "control" through this behavior.

Overeaters also cause an increase of enkephalin through satiation with food, especially "pleasant" tasting foods. As stresses increase, they realize that if they eat excessively, they return to calm – via enkephalin release.

People who crave chocolate may feel less than special, unloved. If they binge on chocolate, they provide the brain with phenylethylamine, which is our "love" chemical. When PEA is available, we feel special.

The trauma of codependency lowers enkephalin and GABA availability. Family members feel increasingly anxious, unworthy, and helpless as a result. Seeking to fill this void of inadequacy, they substitute the norepinephrine and dopamine rush achieved by doing more, being more, and taking charge, much as "workaholics" attempt to do. With the increasing conversion of dopamine to norepinepherine more and more dopamine is depleted and the "co-dependent" begins to sense less love and attachment to significant others.

To a significant degree, compulsive behaviors can be explained neurochemically. Once you come to understand and utilize this knowledge it all begins to make sense.

Alterations in the balance of brain chemistries alters our thoughts, feelings, and behaviors. People with well balanced brain chemistry not only appear enviable assertive, confident, in control, concerned for others, and able to think quickly, but will feel these same capabilities within themselves. It does not occur to them that there is anything to fear, because all systems are in concert and their survival does not appear threatened. They are able to take life as it presents itself and alter their thoughts and behaviors to feel comfortable. They have no need for external chemical input. Alcohol, other drugs and destructive behaviors present a destabilizing influence to them. They sense chemicals as "dope". But people who gain positive feelings from chemicals and other compulsions, in spite of adverse effects, may think of these chemicals and behaviors as "hope".

As the famed psychologist Abraham Mazlow has shown us, the foundation for building toward self-actualization must be physical stabilization. This stabilization in chemical dependency and freedom from destructive compulsive behaviors must involve improving brain chemistry capabilities. In the past we have attempted to construct the second, third , and fourth levels of a self-esteem "building" without providing a sound physiological foundation. As a result, the structure often collapses.

To wage an effective war on alcohol, other drugs and dysfunctional compulsive behaviors, we must make "peace" with our biochemistry.

CHAPTER 7

Chemical Susceptibilities

We can think of chemical susceptibilities existing in three categories: "Arousal seeking, the joy of fear", "Satiation or calm seeking" and "Mental excursions as in day dreaming", as described by Milkman and Sunderwirth in their informative book "Craving for Ecstasy".

"Arousal Addicts and Addictions" – "The Joy of Fear". These persons seek experiences which increase the release of dopamine and norepinepherine in the brain. They seek to increase the stimulatory impact of transmitters from things such as cocaine, methamphetamine, any "speed" drug. They also are prone to be involved in behaviors which produce risk to their survival such as confrontation, fast driving, "bungy jumping", parachuting, rock climbing without safety harness, gambling excessively and without regard to consequences, shop lifting and increased illegal actions which gain them a "RUSH" of dopamine and adrenalin. When they do these things they tell us they feel "normal". This is due to a lack of stimulatory activity in various areas of the brain which is moved to more "normal" activity level by these actions. The problem with these behaviors, other than the obvious social problems, is that they quickly deplete these chemicals while at the same time diminishing the needed calming chemistries used during normal life activities for effective life management. As dopamine and adrenalin are depleted they sense "no pleasure in life" except when they undertake the various activities that force the release of remaining dopamine, for example. However, as dopamine is depleted it takes more and more "risky" behavior to cause this release of diminishing stores of the transmitter and the person becomes involved in more and more desperate attempts to move out of this "depressed" state and goes deeper and deeper into dependency and addiction.

The first step in overcoming these problems is, obviously, stopping the use of the chemicals or actions causing the problems. Unfortunately this leaves the person with a severely depleted set of brain chemistries which they are unwilling and incapable of living with. This severely depleted state results in "craving" for relief, and what does that best for them at this time – use of the drug or behavior. Therefore, the next step is to immediately begin the replacement of depleted transmitters using the "precursor loading" approach proven thru research to quickly aid in the replacement of dopamine and adrenalin via amino acid and vitamin intake. By taking in the particular building blocks for depleted chemistries provided by NGI's NeuReplenish, for example, the "arousal addict" will begin to sense some relief from the "depression" within a few days and within approximately 90 days on the required regimen will find he or she no longer is seeking the drugs or compulsive behaviors.

Using the supplement is essential to success but only the first of several things to do in the march toward sanity. These persons must avoid all contact with persons, places or things they previously associated with in any using or compulsive behavior situations. Contact with any previous "memory" of use from their past will result in an immediate and intense "craving" for the experience again.

Next they must begin to put a structure and discipline in their lives to deal with everyday problems. Problems and trauma (stress) cannot be ignored but must be dealt with as they arise or the brain will revert to those "cravings" for relief previously achieved by drugs, etc. A person must begin to take care of themselves as other healthy persons do; eat right, get your rest, become a functional human being. After the first 90 days these persons can change to an NGI product called "NeuBecalmd" for ongoing maintenance of brain chemicals necessary for meaningful and effective life management. The structure and discipline must remain or "relapse" will occur and each time recovery becomes more difficult.

"Arousal addicts" must also be careful how often and how strenuous they exercise. Everyone tends to think that if they "exercise" a great deal they will get better sooner. The opposite is true. When they exercise strenuously and raise their heart rate to the same level associated with previous drug use or problem behaviors they will immediately experience a "craving" for their "drug of choice". In addition, when dealing with these persons in a counseling setting it is vital that the counselor be assertive in their actions. Arousal addicts respond to confrontive actions and are repulsed by "laid back", soft spoken advice. If you want an arousal prone person to respond positively it requires an almost "get in your face" approach, or they will take control.

"Satiation prone" addictions are those associated with alcohol, marijuana, anorexia, overeating, tranquilizers, the "**chemistries of contentment**".. These people seek to reduce the negative impact of information coming into their brains from society and internally. Very low self worth (enkephalin deficiency) is a common denominator as well as a chronic sense of "anxiety" from no discernable source. Alcohol reduces anxiety by its' impact on GABA complex activity, impact on opioid activity and general suppression of brain activity. Thru these actions the brain "slows" down and senses less threat from the environment and our internal sense of diminished self concept is improved.

Again, the first step toward recovery for these persons is removal of the drug, including alcohol, or stopping the satiating behavior such as overeating in times of trauma or stress.

Immediate use of the NGI product "NeuRecover" will quickly

begin the repair of deficient brain chemistry to aid in the quest for normal feelings. Again the person must follow the same principles described earlier, avoid previous people, places or things associated with the dependency, put structure and discipline into their life management, address problems promptly, eat well, and basically take quality care of themselves. These actions along with the supplement "NeuRecover" will, in these first 90 days, help tremendously in the recovery effort. After 90 days the product "NeuBecalmd" can be used effectively for ongoing and long term maintenance. Because there is usually a strong genetic component associated with these deficiencies it may be necessary for a person to use the supplement ongoing to maintain a balanced brain chemical capacity.

Satiation prone individuals recoil from confrontation. A counselor must approach them in a firm but supportive manner. They will engage in planning for their recovery if they do not feel that the counselor is looking down on them. Marijuana dependent persons make many "plans" to achieve great results. The problem is their brains have been impacted by the accumulation of delta nine tetrahydrocanabinol (THC) and the actions needed to actually achieve change are disrupted. They make plans but can't seem to "get around to doing" anything about the problem. When you overload a marijuana addict with tasks to accomplish you will lose him/her because the stress of too many expectations will cause their brain chemistry to call for "calming" and their drug is what will do it immediately. Structure and discipline to the structure is the key to recovery for satiation prone individuals. "Facts are Friendly", "What you worry about most is what you must confront next" are the keys to reducing the fear of all the problems around them. I always said I thought I could "diagnose" dependencies with these types of individuals if I could find out if they open their mail daily or if they try to avoid it. The "fear of the unknown" is their biggest relapse figure.

"Mental Excursions" refer to the use of things such as video games, excessive TV, or extended day dreaming to escape the reality of life issues and achieve some sense of calm. Playing video games, watching TV will increase the release of Serotonin since it is the primary sensory input neurotransmitter. With increased Serotonin activity the person senses a more calm, balanced state and many use these actions to do just that. If playing excessive video games or watching TV begins interfering with quality of life then it is an issue that should be dealt with. These people respond to calm, ongoing verbal communications. Very much like the approach with psychedelic drug users – we "talk them down from their fantasy". Using the NGI product NeuBecalmd will contribute the building blocks for those chemistries required for a calm, balanced brain, including the building block for Serotonin.

CHAPTER 8

The Chemical Component to Thoughts, Feelings. & Behaviors

For every thought, every feeling, every behavior there is a neurochemical component in the brain which produces the thoughts, feelings and behaviors. These neurochemicals are called neurotransmitters and they work to interact with specialized brain cells in various parts of the brain and body. Over the years researchers have focused on rather narrow areas of interest and produced their research information on this narrow focus. This is how research is done, and it must be specific and replicable to be valid. Candace Pert and others in the 60's were searching for chemicals that were naturally occurring in us but were producing effects similar to opiate drugs. When a person uses an opiate one of the effects is a profound sense of well being, sense of internal calm, a sense of self-esteem. During this work they found and named natural transmitters which could also achieve this effect and named them "enkephalins" (in the head). Later endorphins were described and soon all of these chemicals were generally being referred to as "endorphins", although this is not completely accurate.

As I read this research I wondered if somehow I was deficient in these chemicals and could this be the reason I felt no sense of "completeness"? If so, why was I deficient and could it be corrected? I recalled that at various times I had been prescribed "pain medications" from a physician and remembered that in fact when I took them I really felt "better". Not just relief from some physical pain but relieve from the psychological pain of inadequacy.

ADDICTION

To many, the word **addiction** is only used for losers. It is a direct implication that an individual is lazy, weak-willed and has questionable morals. This is simply not the case.

Our brain's job is to process information and keep us alive; it is the command center of the body. But, it has to have the right neurochemicals to function properly. These neurochemicals are made from the foods we eat (or drink), the nutritional supplements we take, and the process of synthesis. When our brain is functioning as it was created to function, it has the correct balance of neurons for sending and receiving, and the reuptake for reuse procedure works as it should. Everything is balanced and harmonious.

But, the brain is very frugal and will not expend the time or energy to internally produce a chemical that it does not perceive it needs to produce. Therefore, if necessary chemicals are provided externally (by whatever source or activity), the brain will not only allow this, but will even grow to depend on the external chemical source.

The brain does not distinguish bad chemicals from good chemicals, or bad chemical sources from good chemical sources. It only knows chemicals. Chemical sources can be from prescription drugs used wisely, prescription drugs used unwisely, street drugs, alcohol, nicotine, caffeine, etc. Neurochemicals are also produced or depleted through certain activities.

Physical dependence develops when an individual is exposed

to an external chemical source at a high enough dose for long enough that the body adapts and develops a tolerance for the [drug]. This means that higher doses are needed to achieve a drug's original effects. If the person stops taking the drug, uncomfortable symptoms associated with the chemical withdrawal will occur.

Psychological dependence can also develop-a belief that we must have the chemicals to function.

Craving is the result of the brain imprinting a pleasurable, even euphoric, memory in association with the external source of a particular chemical. The subconscious memory then motivates the individual to seek this source because of the false imprint. The brain, in effect, has been trained that using the drug (or external chemical source) is the fastest way to achieve that euphoric feeling. This learning process then produces a new appetite or drive to seek the source of that wonderful feeling. An addiction has developed.

This craving or addiction is most often activated by a memory of pleasure. When we feel unhappy, our brain will flash a picture for us of the last time we felt happy. It will show us exactly where we were, who we were with, and what we were doing (eating, ingesting, drinking, smoking, viewing, etc.) to feel that rush of enjoyment or gratification.

Because the brain has sensed that a certain chemical is being supplied externally (from whatever source), it will slow down its internal production of that chemical. Therefore, when the chemical is needed, the brain activates the slide show.

Also, when we are in a situation with people or places in which a previous activity or pattern of drug use has been established, those desires to "feel good" will return with a vengeance – slide show re-runs in living color.

Addictions are chemical complications brought on by a number of things. Decisions that have been made, knowingly or unknowingly, that cause our brain to stop internally producing crucial neurochemicals are the foundations for positive reinforcement by outside chemicals. If chemical cravings and dependencies are left unchecked, people, places, activities and lifestyles that once brought normal pleasures, suddenly do not fit in with the [drug] use. Often the heavy drug user will actually come to resent people or lifestyles that do not fit in with that drug use. A dependence on the immediate, fast, predictable chemical source has developed. The brain has shut down its internal production in favor of the external source that has been provided.

Addictive behaviors or substances can mimic the action of chemicals the brain produces to send messages of pleasure to the brain's reward center and produce an artificial feeling of pleasure by chemically acting like certain normal brain messenger chemicals (neurotransmitters). Interests in and the motivation to make life's normal rewards work are "short circuited."

The neurotransmitters that are generally affected are the opioids, dopamine, norepinephrine, GABA and serotonin.

It is imperative that responsible steps be taken to provide the brain with the fuel to once again make the neurochemicals internally. As internal production returns to normal, the cravings for external sources will become more manageable and may subside altogether for many.

The best way to accomplish this is to make the lifestyle changes you can. Such as develop new friendships, improve diet and exercise routines, drink plenty of fresh water and take nutritional supplements that contain vitamins, minerals and amino acids. Amino acids are the precursors for building neurochemicals naturally.

CHAPTER 9

ADD/ADHD ---- MAYBE NOT

For the last 15 years or so the "ADD/ADHD" label has been the popular medical description attached to a number of difficult symptoms appearing, especially, in school age children. These symptoms include, among others, distractibility, difficulty in focusing, fidgeting, generally paying attention to the surroundings rather than the task at hand, especially as it related to male students. The female "problem" students would also display distractibility but would then tend to withdraw and were often "labeled" dissociative, another medical cubby hole. Because the females would be less disruptive, overall, the males received the majority of the focus.

Distinctive medical research published by Dr. Bruce Perry, MD, PhD, and his team, brought exacting new light to this problem BUT has been largely ignored by the overall medical and societal communities. The most likely reason for this exclusion is the overwhelming amount of literature furnished by large drug companies invested in medications addressing this "excitability".

What if the initial label of "ADHD" is not quite accurate? What if we have been overlooking an even more serious situation in the brains of these children, and young adults? What if we fail to properly address pointed issues in these developing brains, and minds? The result may well be a generation or more of adults with untreated brain chemistry problems which may set them up for ongoing serious difficulty dealing with life issues presented to them, as they are presented to us all.

Drawing extensively from Dr. Perry's work we need to become aware of the actual happenings in the developing brains of young children. First, we must realize that children are not particularly "resilient" in the face of turmoil and trauma. They do not just "bounce back" from stress and worry presented in the struggling family. Even though they may be unable at the early age to understand the intricacies of all the issues confronting survival by the family their brain "knows" that a threat is present, picks up the stress and tension in the environment, and goes about what it is supposed to do to ensure survival. It aggressively programs a "fight or flight" response into the areas of the brain necessary for survival.

In addition, the "memories" of all the sensory issues related to the trauma are captured for ongoing reference as they mature when similar environmental events "line up" with previously stored patterns of previous threats to survival. This means that anything we see, hear, smell, taste, or touch that triggers similar brain chemistry patterns associated with previous trauma will AUTOMATICALLY initialize a "fight or flight" response, even though the current surroundings may have no relation to a real threat. When the brain is in a "fight or flight" mode, especially in males, there is no "sitting still, focus on what is in front of you" for the individual so programmed. Sitting still means "danger may overtake us, may be fatal".

In the case of the female student confronted with some aspect of sensory input that mirrors any trauma she may have experienced as a young child she initially exhibits a "startle" response (looking around excitedly, not focused on what is in front of her) and then, due to a release of opioid brain chemicals, she "turns inward" to a more calm, safe, setting in her mind. This has allowed the females to survive in the face of life threatening events from the earliest "cave man groups" and ensured the survival of the species. Today we mistakenly "label" this young female student "dissociative" and attempt to medicate her for more appropriate interaction in her surroundings. How sad.

Sad because we are not incorporating the valid understandings of what may actually be happening but force our next generations to be overmedicated.

What if these children had been exposed to the worry and strife of families trying to survive today? What if their survival had been threatened with the loss of a home to foreclosure (which they would not understand but would still experience)? What if these children had been exposed to fighting between parents, physical abuse by one parent or the other? What if these children had been exposed to arguments about how to pay the bills, how to buy enough food, how to get new clothes and shoes? What if these children had been exposed to parents discussing the loss of jobs, or the likelihood of separation or divorce? Do you suppose any or all of these issues would be construed by their developing brain as "threats to survival"? OF COURSE THEY WERE!

As these children grew they became more and more aware of the constant threats around them and, each time one of these threats lined up with previously stored patterns associated with recollections of trauma, they were automatically put under the chemical influence associated with survival. As Dr. Perry has said, "these children became constantly "hypervigalent". Constantly scanning their surroundings for threat, always ready to run or fight, withdrawing into their own safe, internal world. These reactions were appropriate in certain situations but not "appropriate" in a classroom setting. The problem was these children received sufficient sensory input, something they heard, saw, smelled or touched, that triggered automatic reactions over which they had no control.

Many of us have experienced, and many have observed, some people reacting aggressively when their brains received sensory input reminding them of threatening situations they had faced. Women who have been attacked have been seen to recoil in situations when they hear, see, or smell something that triggers memory of the trauma, even though the current situation has nothing to do with the traumatic event. Women have told us that when this happens they are able to "retreat in their minds to a safe place", just as they did during the traumatic initial event. So we say they have become "dissociative". SAD

I vividly recall an instance during a treatment group I was leading in outpatient alcohol/drug treatment. This was a small group of 6 individuals which included one young woman. As the group went around introducing themselves I saw this young lady "recoil" when one of the men starting talking. She slumped in her chair and I could actually see her pupils constrict almost instantly. I was careful not to mention this during group but at the conclusion pulled her aside and let her know what I had observed. She said "when Mark started talking it sounded exactly like the guy who had raped me at knife point" What had happened was that this new sensory input had lined up with previously stored patterns of this traumatic memory and had immediately alerted her brain that a threat was present. Her brain released Norepinepherine as she was "startled" and then flooded her brain with opioids that allowed her to turn inward to a more calm and safe "place". The opioids also caused the constricting of her pupils, just as opiate drugs do. When I explained all this to her she was dramatically relieved, and it also gave us information for further counseling efforts.

Many soldiers returning from combat tell us that when they "hear" a helicopter they immediately get ready to run. During their time in combat the sounds of helicopters could have been supportive or threatening, depending on where they were.

It is time we move toward correctly identifying possible situations for these children, and adults, which bring about the distractibility et al now labeled "ADD/ADHD" and seek to deal with the real problem issues and brain chemical difficulties. These persons most likely are suffering the long lasting effects of various stressful events and should be approached entirely differently than current "labeling". If we just become aware of what has likely happened, work to help these children and adults acknowledge and then dampen these traumatic memories, as well as help repair the brain chemistry depleted by the stress and trauma, they can overcome these issues and interact appropriately.

NeuroGenesis, Inc. has, for years now, provided nutritional supplements formulated specifically to help with deficiencies caused by trauma and stress. This pre-cursor loading of specific amino acids, vitamins and minerals, has been shown to improve the diminished calming chemistries, help with overall balance of the chemistry associated with trauma and loss and allow the individual to more effectively deal with the situation confronting them. Studies done by scientists at NGI, and others, have validated the fact that trauma and stress dramatically depletes the chemistries necessary to allow the individual to remain calm and focused during stressful times.

NeuBecalmd, for instance, has been used since the mid 1980's and post respective reports by consumers as well as health care providers incorporating this in their arsenal of treatment approaches have validated that helping rebuild lost chemistry though proper supplementation does indeed work.

CHAPTER 10

Nicotine Addiction

The first thing nicotine does in the brain is to facilitate the release of norepinephrine, and the person feels a lift in energy. The second thing nicotine does is fill and activate certain acetylcholine receptor sites necessary for concentration and memory. The third thing that happens is that acetaldehyde in the smoke combines with dopamine and produces salsolinol, which fills and activates enkephalin sites, and the person senses an increased sense of well being. With a chronic release of norepinephrine, we begin to lose GABA as well as enkephalin, and the person feels increased anxiety when attempting to quit smoking abruptly.

When a person attempts to stop smoking, he or she experiences: (1) a loss of the energy due to the reduced release of norepinephrine by nicotine, (2) an inability to concentrate and think abstractly due to an acetylcholine deficiency produced by the replacement of acetylcholine with nicotine, and (3) anxiety and a sense of incompleteness due to limited availability of GABA and enkephalin.

To put it simply, smoking energizes you, helps you concentrate and keeps you calm. Try to quit – you have no energy, you can't think and you feel anxious.

45

In conclusion, alterations in the balance of brain chemistry alter our thoughts, feelings and behaviors. People with well-balanced brain chemistry appear enviably assertive, confident, in control, concerned for others and able to think quickly. Because all systems are in concert, their survival does not appear threatened. They are able to take life as it presents itself and alter their thoughts and behaviors to feel comfortable. There is no need for external chemical input. Nicotine and other drugs present a destabilizing influence to them.

Maslow has shown us the foundation for building toward self-actualization must be physical stabilization. The stabilization must involve improving brain chemistry capabilities. Today nutritional supplement combinations are available that dramatically enhance neurotransmitter availability and hasten the recovery to acceptable, comfortable, positive feelings and thoughts.

In the past, we have attempted to construct the second, third and fourth levels of self esteem building without providing a sound physiological foundation. As a result, the structure often collapses. To wage an effective war on nicotine, we need to make peace with our neurochemistry.

CHAPTER 11

Beacons Of Compulsive Behavior

"In the drama of human excess we are compelled by repetitious urges to become energized, to relax, to imagine. These areas of consciousness are the beacons of compulsive behavior that came to be known and described as "addictions". Prior to the 1960's "addiction" was used only to describe the abusive use of alcohol and other drugs. Gradually addiction came to imply psychological need, over and above the traditional constructs of physical demand and distress upon withdrawal." (Milkman and Sunderwurth)

By the early 1970's the concept of addiction was further extended to include non-intoxicating substances, so that smoking and eating were widely accepted as addictive behaviors. Compulsion, loss of control, and continuation despite harmful consequences became new criteria for the determination of addiction. Furthermore, the notion of a "drug of choice" suggested that some individuals would become harmfully involved with only some substances, depending on their specific needs. This implied that despite the inherent pleasure-inducing properties of certain drugs, only a proportion of those who experimented would slip into a pattern of compulsive use. Moreover, not only did people react differently to the same drug, but the same person might display entirely different patterns of use or abuse at various times of life.

This awareness then has led us to a more sophisticated, realistic definition of addiction: "Addiction is a compulsive, chronic, progressive, potentially fatal biochemical process which has nothing to do with character or willpower." (T. Neher, 1990)

It is unnecessary to develop separate sets of principles to explain how drug use and other compulsive behaviors gain control over human life. Drugs, food, sex, gambling, and aggressive episodes all give prompt, salient, and short-lasting relief to the people who indulge in them. In addition to sharing pleasure-inducing properties, both substance use and other mood-altering activities tend to produce an initial state of euphoria, which is then followed by a negative emotional state; that is, a high followed by a low.

A two stage model for the origins and progression of addictions includes: the acquisition phase in which the novice begins and continues a potentially compulsive activity because of pleasurable sensations brought about through the experience. The environment where the desired feeling occurs becomes associated with a "rush" or sense of pleasurable well-being. The human body eventually adapts to most novel stimulation by reducing the potency of its effect. The user or performer soon needs more of the mood-altering activity in order to experience similar alterations in feeling. The addicted climber must increasingly seek out more difficult cliffs, and the hooked sky diver compulsively finds more challenging and frightening drops. In the maintenance stage of addiction, a person is no longer motivated by a sense of pleasure from the need-gratifying behavior. Rather, the repetitive activity now serves only to relieve the sense of despair and physical discomfort that is felt when the mood-altering actions or substance is not present.

Loss of control and progressive deterioration of social, economic, or health functions have emerged as the familiar course of human compulsion. Treatment techniques for a variety of habitual problem behaviors have thus become increasingly modeled after widely publicized drug and alcohol intervention approaches. Gamblers

Anonymous, Overeaters Anonymous, and Sexaholics Anonymous are contemporary treatment organizations that rely heavily on the twelve-step recovery process originally developed by Alcoholics Anonymous. These organizations provide a safe and positive setting and a set of behaviors designed to help the individual put structure and discipline into their lives to offset the compulsions of addiction.

Addiction is evident when one becomes progressively unable to control the beginning or end of a need-fulfilling activity. Yet below the surface of this descriptive formulation are more profound explanatory links. These seemingly unrelated "newly discovered" addictions are actually connected by biochemical threads only recently identified and clarified. Compulsive problem behavior is solely the responsibility of the brain and its' hundred billion or so nerve cells or neurons communicating with each other through trillions of interconnections. This "talking" is referred to as neurotransmission, and its language is chemistry. From a purely biochemical standpoint, neurotransmission controls all emotions, perceptions, and bodily functions. In other words, for every thought, every feeling and every action there is a neurochemical configuration producing it. If we lose a hand or a foot, we are still recognized as the same person, but if our synaptic chemistry changes dramatically we seem to possess altogether different personalities.

Scientists have not yet been able to identify just how many neurotransmitters are in use by the brain and body, but it is likely in the hundreds. Of this number less than 20 have been identified as to structure and function. Among those identified Dopamine, Serotonin, GABA and the Opioids (met-enkephalin in particular) appear to play a major role in many aspects of normal life activities as well as in those compulsive behaviors which become detrimental to human life.

CHAPTER 12

A Brief Description of Neuronal Systems

A brief description of neuronal systems helps to understand the roles and effects of various neurotransmitters: the brains neurons are composed of three basic parts; the cell body which contains the nucleus and other organelles, dendrites which receive impulses from other neurons, and axons which carry impulses away from the cell body. The cell body acts as a small computer. It must decide from a "discussion" with a multitude of surrounding neurons whether to "fire" and send the impulse to the axon, or to remain dormant. Firing either occurs or it does not. It is an "all or nothing" principle. There are no weak or strong impulses; all impulses are of the same magnitude. The intensity of "feeling" is determined by the frequency of neuronal firing rather than by "strength" of the electrochemical jolt.

One of the more interesting facts about the brain is that it is not "hard-wired". The brain has no physical contacts among it trillions of interconnecting neurons. Each nerve cell is physically separated from the other billions of nerve cells by a small space called a "synapse". When the cell body "fires" the impulse travels down the long fiber of the axon to the synapse separating the axon of one neuron from the dendrites of another. The impulse is carried across the synapse to the receiving neuron by small molecules that are released into the synapse. These molecules, known as neurotransmitters, move across the synapse and attach themselves to sites known as receptors, which are embedded in the membrane of the postsynaptic terminals of the dendrites.

The receptors are tailor made to receive only neurotransmitters that have a shape that complements that of the receptor. This relationship between neurotransmitter and receptor is very much like a lock and key. Just as only a key with the correct shape will work in a given lock, only those neurotransmitters with the right shape will activate the specific receptors designed for them. If a sufficient number of receptors on the postsynaptic membrane become occupied by neurotransmitters, there is a change in the electrical balance of this membrane that results in a transfer of the impulse from the presynaptic neuron to the postsynaptic neuron.

As soon as the neurotransmitter does its job it is released from the receptor back into the synapse where it is usually taken back into the pre-synaptic (sending side) neuron where it can be reused. If it is not taken back it may be broken down by enzymes or taken away into the glia for use in other functions. This "reuptake" process is very important to maintain supplies of transmitter for ongoing activity.

Just as it is possible to put keys of slightly different shapes into a given lock, it is possible to introduce into the synapse molecules with shapes similar to neurotransmitters that will attach to the receptor sites. However, these pseudo-neurotransmitters do not change the electrical balance of the postsynaptic membrane, and in fact block the receptor sites from receiving neurotransmitters that transfer the nerve impulse. This action prevents the receiving neuron from initiating an impulse and thus "blocks" the normal activity.

This is the reasoning behind the use of certain drugs, for instance, used in the treatment of mental disorders. The current hypothesis surrounding Schizophrenia is that, for some reason not yet fully understood, excessive amounts of the neurotransmitter

Dopamine are released from the presynaptic (sending) neurons in multiple areas of the brain at the same time. This excessive release occupies, and triggers, impulses in multiple areas at the same time. This action then may initiate "voices" or "sights" or "sounds" or "actions" in multiple areas of the brain at the same time.

These multiple and varied firings of the neurons are sensed by the effected individual as real and their response often is seen as the evidence of "multiple personalities". This excessive, simultaneous firing of neurons can be controlled with the introduction of "fake" neurotransmitters in the form of the drug Haldol, for instance. This molecule has a configuration very similar to the molecule Dopamine. Haldol will fill the receptors but will not energize or activate the postsynaptic neuron because it is not the correct "key" for this lock. Blocking these neurons from firing multiple times in multiple areas allows the individual to more normally experience the environment and respond in more normal ways.

Until the cause, or causes, of this condition are determined, the most effective, and beneficial, method of treatment is to treat the symptoms of the condition with medications blocking excessive firing.

Chapter 13

The Function Of Dopamine

Dopamine appears to have multiple functions in various parts of the brain and body. For the purposes of dealing with "addiction" the impact of dopamine, or the loss of dopamine, will be confined to some of the functions identified in the brain. For the purposes of this writing we can consider Dopamine functioning in areas of the brain having to do with "reward and pleasure", "love and attachment", "excitement and commitment", and "altruism" (an unselfish concern for the well-being of others).

It appears that addiction can form from either of two sets of circumstances or a combination of both. A person can be born with a deficiency of a certain (or various) neurotransmitters (genetic susceptibility) or develop a deficiency through the impact of a traumatic environment. In other words, for a dependency to develop there must first exist or be developed a shortage of normal neurotransmitter function which can then be influenced by the ingestion of specific chemicals or by the undertaking of certain behavioral actions.

In the case of stimulant drugs or excitatory behaviors the primary targets are the neurons normally receiving dopamine molecules to initiate a "rewarding or pleasurable" response.

Consider genetic susceptibility first. We get half our genes from mom and half from dad, and we don't get a choice. If a combination of the genetic factors defining the availability of dopamine produce a low level, or less than adequate level of this transmitter, then those areas of the brain utilizing dopamine will not function or produce the optimum "feeling" or emotional state required for normal experience. A dopamine deficiency, from whichever source, will result in the individual having difficulty experiencing pleasure from normal human interaction. This person will seldom experience the "reward" of experiences usually thought to be rewarding by society. With a deficiency of dopamine this individual will not be able to experience the human emotion we refer to as "love" or attachment, even for his or her own children or other family members. For a dopamine deficient person life is not colorful or particularly fulfilling. He/she does not experience or express pleasure or reward from human interaction as experienced by others. In other words this person does not feel "happy" with life. He/she becomes aware that somehow they are "different" than others they may interact with. If the opioid chemistries were deficient the individual would always feel "less than, unworthy, insecure." This genetically influenced person experiences this negative set of chemistry from birth.

What about the person who is born with sufficient dopamine and the opioids but eventually becomes dopamine and enkephalin deficient? This occurs as the result of the person living in a state of chronic environmental trauma (stress). "Stress" has been identified as a human condition for almost a hundred years. However, it is only recently that the full extent of the impact of chronic traumatic events has been scientifically studied. It is true that we react quicker and with focus if some minimal stress is present during a situation. This is positive and necessary for resolution of potentially threatening situations. But, if the "threat" is not quickly resolved, there is a price to pay and a major component of the price is a depletion of dopamine and the enkephalins. How does this happen? When faced with a threat, any situation which seems to potentially threaten our survival, the brain releases noradrenalin to prepare to run or fight. This is a normal, human mechanism meant to help insure our survival as a species. In the past "threats to survival" were thought to be the more extreme physical threats or situations in which our very life seemed threatened. We now know there is a much more insidious aspect to human trauma.

Everyday human existence is laced with "threats to our survival". The major "stressor or trauma" in the vast majority of American lives is financial. This trauma is acute and chronic at the same time. As we face this extreme and ongoing "threat to our survival" the brain releases more and more noradrenalin to either run from or fight off the threat. Noradrenalin is made from Dopamine. As more and more dopamine is depleted to supply the fight or flight response we become increasingly "depressed". We sense less pleasure, less love and attachment for family members, less concerned about the well being of others and increasingly focused on our personal survival. Since long standing noradrenalin release requires the use of enkephalin to stay in balance the calming opioids, enkephalins, are also depleted and a sense of inadequacy is the result.

At this point it would make little difference if we were genetically deficient in dopamine or depleted due to trauma. If, at this point, we for any reason tried cocaine for instance, we would experience an immediate change and relief from the dopamine deficient "depressed" state. Cocaine would immediately block the reuptake of the little dopamine available and force it to stay in the synapse longer. As it remained in the synapse it would immediately fit back into its receptors and produce the limited but now more intense, sense of pleasure. The transmitter would be released back into the synapse but again prevented from being taken backup for storage by the cocaine molecules blocking the reuptake access. This cocaine would remain in place for anywhere between 30 minutes and an hour before being broken down by enzymes and removed. In the meantime the dopamine forced to remain in the synapse would be exposed longer to those enzymes designed to break it down or it would be carried away into other parts of the brain.

When the dopamine can finally get back into presynaptic (sending) neurons for reuse there is even less than there was before the cocaine. Now, as it is released to fill receptor sites there is even less activation of the "pleasure" centers than before the cocaine and the brain will IMMEDIATELY respond by requesting more of the substance which "helped" it work before. This "craving" is intense, immediate, and undeniable. The "state of mind" resulting from this extreme loss of dopamine is a state which is not possible to ignore. The "depression" is so deep, so dark, so full of anguish that the user will start to immediately seek a source of another "fix". If another use is indeed accomplished there will be an immediate relief as remaining dopamine is prolonged in receptor sites. BUT, this second use of the drug does not, cannot, produce the same relief or high as the first time because less dopamine is available. It doesn't make any difference to the user though as some relief is better than no relief. And so "addiction is born."

The use of an amphetamine produces basically the same result with the difference being the "high" is not quite as intense but lasts longer as it takes more time for the amphetamine to be removed.

Or, we might have a few drinks of liquor or beer or wine, just to relax. These chemicals would immediately begin the process of "making up for" the deficient calming chemistries and we feel "less depressed or threatened" when we have the drinks. Marijuana, tranquilizers, all "depressant drugs" would do the same and so "addiction is born".

Everyone begins their first use of a substance for one of two reasons, or a combination of the two. The first is "curiosity". "I wonder what it would be like if I did it"? The second is "peer pressure". "Everyone else is doing it why shouldn't I"? It does not make any difference "why" someone starts the use of a substance, it only matters what state their biochemistry is in when they do start.

If a deficiency encounters a substance which seems to improve a state of mind then it is "positive" as far as the brain is concerned. Brain chemistry does not have a value system. Brain chemistry does not know right from wrong or good from bad. It only knows chemistry. It is the combinations of various and multiple chemistries that produce thoughts, feelings and actions that we view as a "value system". Poor or deficient chemical systems express poor or deficient value systems.

As more and more dopamine is depleted from the systems in the brain requiring this transmitter for function we express the effects of the diminished transmitter actions. Scientists at Johns Hopkins have shown us "mappings" of the various transmitter functions. In the frontal lobe of the brain, encompassing cerebral cortex and part of the limbic system, is a small walnut sized area known as "the seat of altruism". Altruism is defined as "the unselfish concern for the well-being of others". In other words, a "social conscience". As dopamine is depleted in this area the person becomes increasingly unconcerned about the well being of others and increasingly focused on personal need.

This same result can occur as a result of prolonged stress or ongoing human traumatic conditions. As the threat to our survival goes on and on we find ourselves caring less and less about others. We find that our "love" for others seems lessened, our decreased attachment to family deepens and we move into a space of personal survival. This happens not because we are "bad" people but because we have lost dopamine availability and function in those areas necessary to perform those functions. Society, however, may tend to label the person "sociopathic" as he/she displays an increasing distain for the well-being of others.

In this dopamine deficient condition it is not necessary to take a substance to effect a change in mind and mood. We have all heard of "go shopping" to "help us feel better". Why does this work? When we "buy" something, especially if it is somewhat out of our reach or need, the brain releases dopamine to initiate an excitement or pleasure response. This physical act will then work to relieve the deficiency somewhat, but only temporarily. But this relief is better than nothing. The individual may take the item home and never even open the box.

The reason is that it is the purchase, not the owning, that releases dopamine and improves mood. So he/she goes back and buys again. Each time it requires the purchase of more or more expensive items to bring about sufficient dopamine action to bring about "pleasure". Many times this "buying" to help the mood becomes "stealing" to get a high of dopamine. Shoplifting, stealing credit cards, selling things to get money to buy, or gamble, will continue to release dopamine. But, like substance use, the dopamine is increasingly diminished and eventually even the most bizarre actions produce little pleasure.

Persons addicted to gambling gamble to bet, not win. Winning may be necessary to continue the process but the primary "rush" and "high" is the bet. More and bigger bets come until the person has to start selling everything they own or have accumulated in savings to try to get that initial rush of dopamine again. It won't happen because it cannot and the person finds themselves losing families and fortunes in an effort to achieve the unachievable. With dopamine depleted, however, they seem to not "care" about others regardless of the relationship.

The reality is they cannot care since they do not possess the transmitters necessary to produce those emotions.

A combination of these deficiencies combined with early and ongoing aspects of trauma during stages of development and into adolescence and adulthood are the foundations for "predatory sexual assaults" so damaging to all involved.

CHAPTER 14

The Impact of Family Trauma

As stated earlier studies done by Bruce Perry, MD, PhD et. al at Baylor University documented the impact of family trauma on very young children. These studies demonstrated that children being raised in an atmosphere of stress, trauma, experienced the same neurochemical depletions as adults. Even though the children could not understand why the family was in such turmoil, around finances for instance, their brains were able to pick up the presence of threat to their survival and their brains began the same neurochemical events and depletions seen in adults. As these children grew and if the trauma remained they showed the same lack of emotional freedom and the same presence of chronic anxiety as adults. Perry and others believe that much of the condition we have come to label as ADHD may well stem from this effect of trauma at a young age. It now appears that children are NOT resilient but are malleable. Their brains grow and develop based on their surroundings.

If not corrected could this early environment be responsible for the increasing numbers of defiant and rebellious young people as they attempt to interact in society with a deficient system intended to help them interact in healthy ways?

Traditional medical interventions for these conditions typically include the use of "antidepressants" intended to relieve the dopamine, and other transmitter, dysfunction. The problem with this as the only approach is that these medications typically work to block the reuptake of transmitters so that they work longer in the hope of relieving the deficient system. The issue is that this was just what the drug or activity was doing to the chemical balances. If taken long enough the medications, in some people, do help the repair process and the eventual return of normal mood. For many they do not and the person is left in the "depressed" state to attempt to function in society.

Following the introduction of a drug known as Prozac, an apparent selective serotonin reuptake inhibitor (SSRI), there were many documented cases of what appeared to be suicide and suicidal ideations in persons diagnosed previously with "depression". The medical community in its desire (and haste) to improve the lives of people "diagnosed" with depression began to routinely prescribe this new family of drugs to persons, many times without in-depth screening and evaluation. An extreme deficiency of the neurotransmitter serotonin results in a person experiencing extreme mood fluctuations, sleep problems, and sensory distortions. Lack of direct sunlight for prolonged periods may be one of the causes of this depletion but more likely it is the presence of chronic, unrelenting trauma (stress) in the persons life.

When the "antidepressant" was administered and blocked the reuptake for reuse of the serotonin molecules they were further depleted by enzymes and/or carried away to be used in other areas. The person now had an even more extreme shortage of this necessary transmitter and the despair became deeper and more prolonged. Many, as a result, decided to end their lives rather than live in this terribly dark and unhappy state.

No one can take a "pill" to solve their problems.

CHAPTER 15

Serotonin And The Monoamines

I mention serotonin here because it is of the same family of chemicals as dopamine, the monoamines. When a drug or behavior impacts one monoamine it also impacts the others to some degree. So now the person taking the "antidepressant" was not only depleting serotonin but also reducing dopamine. The combination of the loss of both of these transmitters is so debilitating that any change from any source is seen as a "gift" and further actions to change this altered state become ingrained.

An example involves a neurotransmitter we all have to some degree called "phenylethylamine". This neurotransmitter serves as our "lust" transmitter so to speak. Phenylethylamine (PEA) is released in response to sensory input from another person. It is what "attracts" us to another in a sensual way. When PEA is released we immediately feel "excited and special".

Consider a person who is dopamine and enkephalin deficient and who encounters a member of the opposite sex (typically but not necessarily) who excites the release of the "depressed" persons PEA. Suddenly they no longer are depressed but feel excited and special. Like any "addictive substance" we quickly become tolerant to the PEA being used to create excitement and a special feeling. We must now seek more personal and intimate relationship interactions to continue the release of PEA, just as a cocaine addict must use more and more of the drug. Soon the PEA will no longer "excite" the person and they sense the relationship has "lost its excitement and meaning."

So they turn to another person to again cause their PEA to function. But this will only work for a short time then they must seek a new relationship to make their PEA function. Because of this neurochemical, and the deficiency of dopamine preceeding, this person goes from relationship to relationship to relationship attempting to feel excited and special.

Many broken hearted persons are left in the wake of this confusing nightmare. However, without sufficient dopamine to elicit a concern nothing will deter this "addict" from further addictive destruction.

No single neurotransmitter functions alone in the myriad of human emotions. Each neurotransmitter has primary functions and primary areas of function. Most neurotransmitters function throughout the body as well as in the brain. Dopamine, however, is one of the most, if not the most important and impactful transmitter we have encountered.

Reward and pleasure are primary forces driving human interaction and existence. When these are unavailable what really is there left to look forward to?

CHAPTER 16

Treat Brain Chemical Imbalance, NOT Symptoms

ANXIETY, a word we hear often but have never really understood what that meant. In the United States we apply labels to various conditions, mental and physical, which we have become accustomed to associating with various symptoms such as "anxiety", "panic", "stress" and "distractibility" to name a few. These labels do nothing to clarify what is actually happening in the brain to "cause" these symptoms. If all we do is receive treatment for the symptoms, and the cause is allowed to remain, then the symptoms will return and so must we for additional medications. This becomes a frustrating cycle of attempts to obtain relieve with questionable results.

If, however, we look at the brain chemical (neurochemical) imbalances which actually are involved then we can take steps to add the nutritional source or the nutritional supplement source to more directly impact the problem. "Anxiety" is the result of inadequate control of adrenalin or noradrenalin (norepinepherine) which, when not adequately controlled by various calming chemistries, results in a constant state of fight or flight to various degrees. This constant "fight or flight" is labeled nervousness, anxiety, and when it reaches a significant level, panic.

The solutions obtained thru the use of "tranquilizing" drugs may temporarily relieve the symptoms but do nothing to help with the cause - depleted neurochemistries such as the GABA complex, the Opioids and Serotonin. In fact, the use of drugs introduced via oral or other sources will, over time, further reduce the availability of our natural calming chemistries. As this depletion continues we find ourselves in need of more and more of the medications, which will eventually make things even worse, and so on.

In our society we tend to describe various unwanted biological, psychological or social symptoms as evidence of "disease" and often seek medications to intervene in these uncomfortable symptoms. A simple explanation of "anxiety" is as follows:

When an individual is facing any situation which the brain senses as threatening our systems automatically prepare a defense to counter the threat. The first thing that happens is that there is increased outpouring of norepinepherine (adrenalin) in the brain and body which alerts us to fight or flee. As this adrenalin continues to be released various chemical systems are utilized to "calm down" the effect of this adrenalin and bring us to a better balance to deal with the trauma.

If the stressor (trauma) continues to confront us these "calming" chemistries are overused and begin to be depleted. As they are depleted the adrenalin becomes more and more dominant. Increased adrenalin results in increased heart rate, increased respiration, increased surveillance of our surroundings, in other words all the things necessary for our body to defend against the threat.

This "hyper-vigilance" is then labeled "anxiety". When we feel "anxious" for no seeable reason it is termed "free floating anxiety".

It is true that we need the correct adrenalin activity level to fully deal with problems and issues that confront us. As long as the adrenalin release helps us accomplish solutions and then is properly withdrawn we are functioning well.

Many times we seek medications to assist with the calming of the adrenalin effect and are given various "tranquilizers" which will reduce the amount of adrenalin output. However, when we use an external drug, of any sort, to assist our internal chemistries there will be a price to pay. As the various parts of our nervous systems use "tranquilizers" we manufacture less and less of our own needed internal chemistries which are supposed to do the calming. This is the way we become "dependent" on medications and other drugs.

A more effective and natural way to overcome these deficiency states is through proper nutrition and nutritional adjuncts. The calming chemistries we all need are manufactured from amino acids derived from protein along with certain vitamins and minerals. Unfortunately, it is very difficult, almost impossible, to raise deficient neurotransmitters by the use of food as the only source for these specific building blocks. Using specific amino acids and associated vitamins and minerals is, however, a very effective way to raise levels of neurotransmitters and overcome the deficiencies created by stress and medication use.

When we effectively address the deficiencies caused by trauma, stress, or medications we become much more capable of positive actions in the management of our lives. By using nutritional sources of the amino acid building blocks for our chemistry we assist, not deplete, the chemistry needed to "slow the flow" of adrenalin and keep the fight or flight response in check. In other words, curb the anxiety. Medications do NOT help build what we need. They, instead, substitute their action for our natural actions which leads to ongoing problems.

CHAPTER 17

Benzodiazepine (Tranquilizer) Addiction

Understanding this terrible dependency, protracted withdrawal, and successful freedom from the use of tranquilizers is best understood if approached from several fronts.

First: how a dependency develops. Every thought, every feeling, every action we as humans experience requires the interaction of various neurotransmitter systems within our brains. Neurotransmitters are chemicals that interact with receptors in our brains to produce these thoughts, feelings and actions. In the case of tranquilizer drugs, there are two neurotransmitters that are important to understand.

This is neither a complete list of neurotransmitters nor of their functions. However, it can serve as a foundation for understanding what has happened to you and why it is so difficult to "just stop" the use of tranquilizers.

The most important neurotransmitters in this issue are the GABA complex transmitters. They keep things on an even keel, maintain calm, allow rational thoughts and feelings, and keep you in balance. Picture now, a large doughnut with a tiny hole in the center of the doughnut. This is how a GABA receptor complex looks through a microscope. Receptors for GABA are arranged near the outer edge of the doughnut in a circle around the doughnut. When GABA binds (hooks onto) these specific receptors it "tightens" the doughnut and enlarges the hole. This allows chloride to enter the cell through the hole. It is this chloride that slows down firings, slows down thoughts and allows calm feelings.

Neurotransmitter	Functions In	Deficiencies Result In
GABAcomplex	Maintaining calm	Anxiety, panic, racing mind,
Enkephalin	Positive self concept, Internal calm	Low self esteem, feelings of inadequacy

In a ring around the "doughnut" and slightly closer to the hole are receptors that attract and attach tranquilizers. When these drugs attach to the receptors they ASSIST GABA in opening the hole and letting chloride in, slowing things down.

Further in, toward the center of the doughnut, are receptors that attach barbiturates, such as Phenobarbital and Seconal. The alcohol molecule from beer, wine or liquor also attaches at these same receptors, which is one reason to NEVER drink alcohol and take sleeping medications because excessive activation of multiple sets of receptors may result in the stopping of respiration (breathing) which is fatal.

What we are concerned with in this writing are the GABA receptors and the next row of receptors utilized by benzodiazepines. When benzo's are used to assist GABA there is less need for large amounts of GABA to be present, and consequently, the brain reduces the available GABA. In addition the normal transmitters used at these receptors are now needed less because of the external drug being used. (These transmitters have never been fully identified because they act and are released so quickly that we have not been able to 'capture' them for examination.) The brain is not wasteful; it will not make what it does not appear to need. Brain chemistry has NO value system. Brain chemistry does not know right from wrong or good from bad. It only knows chemistry. However, our thought processes *are* based upon available brain chemistry. And thus, in the final analysis, poor brain chemistry results in poor value systems.

Over a period of a few weeks using benzo's your GABA and other transmitters are reduced to the point that you MUST use a drug to activate secondary sites, and assist the GABA in opening the chloride channels. As more and more GABA is depleted you must use more benzo's, and so on. This is dependency. You have become dependent on a drug to produce a function of life. If you try to stop the use of the benzo you have no way to open the chloride channels and slow down the firing of adrenaline throughout your body ~ everything races, everything is a threat. You are now in a constant state of flight or fight. No GABA, no calm and no sleep because your brain will not turn off. Under these circumstances, thought becomes negative and threatening with constant anxiety leading to panic.

Scientists working at NeuroGenesis in the 1980's discovered that stress dramatically reduces GABA. the opioids such as Enkephalin, and Serotonin. In fact, in just 30 minutes time laboratory animals placed under stress experienced a 50% loss of GABA and Enkephalin. If these lab animals had sought a physician at the time they would have been given a benzodiazepine to "relieve the stress". As we have described, however, this drug would worsen the problem of GABA availability. Now GABA is not only threatened by stress (trauma) but by a drug that uses secondary receptors and further reduces the need for available GABA. The animals would have become addicted to (dependent upon) the benzo. When the benzo would have been stopped, the animals would have become "berserk" with activity and flight or fight would have become their life until they died of a heart attack or stroke.

Tapering off of the drug is very necessary. It is essential to slowly reduce the use of a benzo so as not to over stimulate the sympathetic nervous system (adrenal system) and cause potential life threatening events. **It is <u>obvious</u> that your prescribing physician should monitor the tapering process.**

However, tapering does not do enough for the repair of the damaged GABA system. This is why the scientists at NeuroGenesis became determined to develop a supplement that would help build GABA and the supporting chemistries of Enkephalin and Serotonin. NeuRelieve provides the building blocks for these neurotransmitters and is the supplement of choice for tranquilizer withdrawal..

The GABA system also requires the presence of sufficient chloride in the blood stream in order to efficiently reduce anxiety. Salt (sodium chloride) is the obvious source of chloride molecules. If you are concerned about salt and blood pressure, we suggest that you use potassium chloride. Most grocery stores carry this as a salt substitute.

The answer to this problem is not simply chemical. You cannot take a pill and have stress go away. It changes your perception and the way that you feel, but does not address the underlying cause which is/are the problem/s of life that lead to the initial reduction of your natural chemistry. It is true, however, that in order to win the war against benzo's you must make peace with your biochemistry. NeuRelieve (from Neurogenesis) will assist with this.

Now, the second front of the attack on this dependency: Each person suffering from this issue must learn, and utilize daily, a problem solving technique to deal with the "stressors" in their lives. There are three main stressors in life today and they are (1) money problems, (2) job problems and (3) relationship problems. The trauma of any or all of these issues will continue to deplete GABA and the supporting calming chemistry Enkephalin. A good way to deal with many problems is to solve each problem separately. A useful problem solving technique follows:

1. What is the problem?
2. Exactly what is causing the problem?
3. What are three alternative solutions for the problem and the possible consequences of each?

4. Choose one alternative and try it for a period of time (about a month).
5. If it works, keep on doing it. If it doesn't work choose one of the other alternatives.

An Example:

1. What is the problem? The problem is that there are too many bills for the money that is available.
2. Exactly what is causing the problem? There are too many credit card bills and not enough salary to pay them.
3. Three alternatives:
   a. Put away the credit cards, contact creditors and make arrangements for payment.
      Consequence: Not going further in debt; developing a plan to pay the bills. Reduced stress.
   b. Get a second job. Consequence: more money to pay on bills.
   c. Do nothing different. Consequence: More stress, more panic, more debt, more problems.
4. Choose one — your decision!
5. Try your solution of choice for 30 days. If things are getting better – keep doing it. If they are not better then choose another solution and try that until you are on a path for relief and success.

You will be unable to get free from tranquilizers and be comfortable if all you attempt is to taper and take pills. You must take charge of your life one issue at a time. If you do not, it will only get worse. Structure and discipline are your allies.

Facts are friendly. Do not avoid information. Get it, deal with it, conquer the problem.

Third Front: When and what you eat!

It is common for persons using tranquilizers to have little or no appetite. When in some stage or phase of withdrawal and adrenaline is pumping and anxiety is high, you have no appetite. (Survival when threatened - run or fight).

You should eat small meals several times a day, if possible. You must provide food for repair of damaged systems. This is no time to "diet". Eat small portions of quality food several times during the day. Avoid caffeine, chocolate, cola drinks (diet or regular) and refined sugar. These substances will add to adrenaline or quickly boost blood sugar that will produce anxiety. You should eat cheese and fruit before bedtime; cottage cheese is best. Use common sense; take care of yourself, and you will recover just fine. Many have done so with complete success.

Continue the use of NeuRelieve daily, up to six per day. If it seems necessary for a larger dose it is safe to do so. It is interesting to note that a drug becomes useless over a period of time for one of three reasons: 1) it becomes toxic, 2) the body becomes use to it so it no longer works, or 3) an allergy to it develops. None of these occur with amino acid adjuncts to therapy, such as NeuRelieve. They are in fact just concentrated, highly nutritional food.

Thirty-days after you have successfully tapered your drug use, and are no longer using any benzo, we suggest you use the supplement BeCalm'd for ongoing support .

Conclusion:

You must win this War on all three fronts: repairing GABA, dealing with the problems, and eating well. There is no other way to be really successful. Taper and take your supplement (NeuRelieve has the building blocks for GABA, Enkephalin, and Serotonin), problem-solve your issues and eat in a healthy manner.

You can do it, *just do it.* Ask yourself if you would like a normal life, with normal issues and normal solutions. If so. then JUST DO IT!

CHAPTER 18

Contributions of Dr. Richard Andrews

Beginning in 1995 I joined Dr. Richard Andrews working with the Seattle/King County Department of Mental Health and Substance Abuse Services. This department was responsible for channeling funds for many, many treatment centers, outpatient and inpatient. The County maintained an inpatient treatment facility which could house about 300 people at any one time. The majority of clients at this center were indigent, many were homeless and all but a very few had no employment. As a consequence of these very difficult factors the use of alcohol and other drugs was their main escape mechanism. Clients were placed at the center for up to 120 days of "treatment". The same people routinely cycled thru the center for "treatment" periodically. The population predictably increased during the winter when cold weather made it more attractive to "go thru it again". I watched as the same men and women came and went over and over, utilizing public funds for the "treatment services" that were expected to help them reenter society as a productive citizen. I decided to test a theory I had about what was not working and why. I began interviewing clients when they had finished the intake process and I ask them all the same questions. (1) What are the major stressors in your life at this time?; and (2)

Were these stressors addressed in a treatment plan? The answer to the first question was, in some order, "I have no place to live", "I have no money", and "I have no job and I don't know how to go about getting a job". The answer to the second question was ALWAYS "NO" these worries were not on their treatment plan.. These men and women ranged in age from 21 to 40 years. When they were ready for discharge (because they had been there the allotted time) I again interviewed them and asked the same questions this way: "Now that you are about to reenter society what are the major worries or stressors in your life?" The answers were just the same as when they started the "treatment". "I don't have a place to live, I have no money and no job". My next question was always "were these concerns addressed in a discharge plan?" The answer, again, was always "NO". At one interview I was talking with an obviously intelligent gentleman and I said this to him; "Describe for me your treatment experience over the last 90 days". He thought for awhile and then said very distinctly "they took away my primary coping tools and left me with all my problems". Isn't that a great use of public funds!!

During this time my immediate supervisor was Dr. Richard Andrews who had been working in the Chemical Dependency Treatment field several years. As I continued searching and researching alternative approaches for recovery services Dick and I became closely aligned with the idea that what had always gone on was not sufficient to prevent relapse after relapse in the population we were supposed to be serving. Dr. Andrews had the amazing capacity to listen to the information I developed, conceptualize it in reference to our client base, outline counselor training courses and set up time lines for the needed training of counselors regarding new approaches to include in their services. Each time he got a training arranged, and we presented it to staff of various centers, we were continually confronted with "that is just too much trouble to integrate into our program". After numerous attempts to assist counselors with new information that was always rebuffed we began to lose energy to continue. It did not take management long to decide to separate us and give each of us an entirely new direction within the County services. Someone once said when they saw Dr. Andrews and I coming thru the doors of their Center with a notebook in our hands "oh gawd here come those terrorists again". Finally the director of our department called me in and said she had heard I was retiring in another year. I acknowledged my intentions to do that and she said "then would you please stop trying to rock the boat and do something else with your time left here. I don't care what you do, just stop telling our agencies they need to change." So, I sat in my cubicle and surfed the net for a year.

CHAPTER 19

The Steps Toward "The Person You Wanted To Be"

The previous description of approaches for problem solving and positive actions are the same approaches that should be incorporated in recovery from any substance or destructive behavior. Once you start to stabilize physiologically you will begin to have the awareness that you are now more safe and secure in your environment. As you continue the correct approaches, including quality nutrition and supplements, you will find yourself actually sensing an attachment and concern, even love, for those around you. Continued positive development will translate internally as an increasing positive self concept, ie. positive self esteem. Just as Mazlow predicted, when we take the correct steps, in the correct order we truly can become the "person we wanted to be". (It is interesting that many of Mazlow's peers said his work would probably not be highly valued until the 21st century. Well, guess where we are at this time.)

However, expecting persons from different backgrounds, different genetics, different traumatic histories, different capabilities, different expectations, to succeed by "going thru the same treatment program" as others in the 'Center' is like fishing and hoping to catch a "steak". Every person must have an individualized treatment plan that incorporates what we have discussed. This is not to say they won't benefit from many 'general discussions' of life problems and solutions. BUT, they must be 'taught' how to manage their lives successfully as individuals in order that they can survive in the ongoing turmoil we call life. This means that persons working as counselors and therapists in the various fields of recovery will need to know how to help their clients with understanding their personal finances, developing budgets, how to create resume's for job seeking, how to problem solve issues in their lives, how to be part of a successful, meaningful relationship. Counselors and therapists should be intimately familiar with mediation and negotiation techniques and be able to help their clients understand the value of effective communication.

In the 1980's and 1990's a man named Terry Gorski started offering continuing education courses for counselors that focused on "Problem Solving Group" approaches. Gorski understood that the major factor in relapse was traumatic life issues that required some form of problem solving before the individual could successfully deal with the difficulties. He published articles and books on "Problem Solving for Relapse Prevention" and shared with hundreds his ideas. Unfortunately only a few agencies adopted and integrated his approaches. If this had become a required adjunct for counselor training we would be miles ahead today in meaningful recovery services. Again, most agencies said "too much trouble to do all that was necessary".

CHAPTER 20

Frustration With "Treatments"
Currently Offered

During numerous discussions with Dr. Andrews it became clear he was increasingly frustrated with "treatment" services offered to perpetrators of physical abuse, particularly sexual abuse. What follows are his words on the subject.

"Common treatment for perpetrators of sexual abuse is first, one of safety. Treatment or therapy is done either in an inpatient (residential) or outpatient setting. The treatment itself generally consists of behavior modification and some form of "talk" therapy, including taking responsibility and practicing empathy. In many cases this approach works and no further such abuse takes place.

More recently, and in my early retirement, I helped intervene for a young teenage boy who had been sexually abusing young boys for a number of years. The juvenile legal system put him on probation requiring that he successfully complete "treatment" at a two year 24-7-365 residential facility which specifically "treated" sexual offender boys between the ages of 12 and 18. This was to be followed by a 2 year probation and on-going outpatient "treatment".

On several occasions, including this boy's treatment intake

process, I became convinced that this young man could not successfully complete the program unless some specific physiological and psychological tests and a comprehensive background information record were completed. That background should have included a conversation or, at least, a perusing of this boy's psychiatric file which included references for need of counseling and aid regarding long term past trauma. IT DID NOT. Why? Because just like most traditional alcohol and drug treatment regimens, full of relapse reports ignored, therapy recommendations for child sexual abuse offenders has its own "blinders" on preventing it from accomplishing the very first goal of any psychological treatment plan: ***evaluate and treat according to INDIVIDUAL DIFFERENCES.***

The clinical staff of this organization was well educated and properly credentialed. But, the facility's adopted treatment regimen was applied to him without investigation into what caused his issues or into the effects these issues were having on his developing brain, not withstanding his behaviors. In the addictions field this "one size fits all" regimen is called "canned or cookie-cutter treatment". After this young man had been in this residential treatment for two years, I was informed by the Clinical Director that the boy was to be kept at the facility for two more months. I asked "what are you going to do differently that hasn't already been done in the previous two years?" His reply was "Oh, we aren't going to do anything differently. The boy will have to do the changing".

I worked for 20 years in various alcohol/drug addiction intervention settings. Treatment centers generally would respond to the likelihood of alcohol/drug relapse with something like "if the clients don't make it this time, maybe they will their **next time** in treatment." One national study on alcohol addiction treatment repetition noted that the seventh time a person went to treatment was likely to be their last. It did not say that by the seventh experience they would be successful just that it was likely their "last". I know the staff I worked with at King County Involuntary

Treatment Center in the late 1990's went to a number of client funerals.

Allow me now to return to the on-going account of the teenage male child offender. He finally leaves the residential facility without "successfully" completing treatment. He goes home, goes back to his previous school and begins outpatient treatment with legal system probation. His problems which brought him to becoming a sexual offender have not been addressed. He has not been "talked out" of re-offending, although he says he would never want to do that again. He's not been "scared straight" by the legal system although he has experienced several depressive states just thinking that he might someday end up in prison. At home and in outpatient treatment, the boy's parents and his counselor note a continuing lack of empathy for nearly everyone. The good behavior he showed at first begins to deteriorate into activities of sexual craving including secret visits to pornographic internet sites (until blocked by parents), stealing pornographic magazines from the neighborhood store and hiding them (until found by parents) and finally sexually abusing a four year old neighborhood child.

He currently is in juvenile prison serving the term which previously had been deferred to allow for "change to occur through treatment".

I believe it prudent, and with a sense of urgency, that we re-visit our current processes of treatment for and prevention of child sexual abuse. I'm ending this chapter quoting Dr. Neher. My own additions (italics are mine) neither diminish his, nor add to it. They only emphasize an on-going tragedy yet unsolved. "To a certain degree compulsive behaviors *(of child sexual abuse offenders)* can be explained neurochemically. To wage an effective war on *(this particular set of)* dysfunctional, compulsive behaviors, we must make peace with our biochemistry".

Dr. Andrews continues to stay in touch with me and we attempt, in the face of reluctance in the treatment fields, to encourage treatment professionals to look at the reality of their efforts.

As for the young man in this scenario I am familiar with his family background and, to a degree, his early childhood experiences. His parents both used various drugs, even in front of him. His early childhood was filled with traumatic threats to survival as drugs, loss of income, injuries and general lack of concern created huge deficiencies of the neurochemicals necessary to think, feel and function normally. The dopamine depletion alone would result in not only diminished pleasure in life but would produce a total lack of empathy for others. He would sense little or no "attachment" to family. Opioid deficiencies resulting from trauma would leave him feeling severely unworthy. Regardless of "why" he first experienced the excitement produced by exercising "power" over a younger child the rush he received from this behavior was immediately and fiercely ingrained in his memory. As he continued to molest he continued to gain short lived excitement and a feeling of being "special", something which never happened in his family environ. Unless he somehow gets access to the necessary physical stabilization and neurochemical rebuilding he will continue to seek unhealthy and illegal activities for the excitement missing in his life.

Child sexual abuse is an "arousal" addiction. The excitement is the result of excessive dopamine release not possible thru normal activity. The product "NeuReplenish" available from Neurogenesis is formulated to specifically address the deficiencies known to be in place in arousal activities. Once the brain is beginning to establish normal activity it is possible for the perpetrator to understand the issues and able to make logical plans to gain normal life skills. Until then we might as well shout into the wind for all the good it will do. They will "tell us what we want to hear" while fantasizing about future activity.

CHAPTER 21

What Is Effective Treatment?

Initial detoxification must be achieved and one of the most effective methods is that promoted by Dr. William Hitt. Centers using his protocol use amino acid, vitamin and mineral formulas introduced into the patient via IV infusion. This intensive supplementation for precursor loading of neurotransmitter building blocks provides a rapid improvement in the levels of depleted neurotransmitters and greatly lessens the chance of intense craving in initial recovery. However, the person must be made aware that ongoing support of the building blocks for needed brain chemistry must be supplemented by products such as made available by Neurogenesis, Inc. Special formulations for specific deficiencies will greatly enhance the physiologic stabilization which Mazlow makes clear must be in place for successful recovery.

Over the last half century "treatment" for chemical dependency has changed little, let alone evolved, even as science made information about addictions more understandable. I read an article given to me several years ago and at that time thought "I need to keep this because it describes the issues in the chemical dependency treatment field exactly". It still does.

"The US standard railroad gauge (distance between the rails) is 4 feet, 8.5 inches. That is an exceedingly odd number. Why was this gauge used? Because that is the way they built them in England, and English expatriates built the US railroads.

Why did the English build them like that? Because the first rail lines were built by the same people who built the pre-railroad tramways, and that's the gauge they used.

Why did 'they' use that gauge then? Because the people who built the tramways used the same jigs and tools that they used for building wagons, which used that wheel spacing.

Why did the wagons have that particular odd wheel spacing? Well, if they tried to use any other spacing, the wagon wheels would break on some of the old, long distance roads in England, because that's the spacing of the wheel ruts.

So---who built those old rutted roads? Imperial Rome built the first long distance roads in Europe (and England) for their legions. The roads have been used ever since.

And the ruts in the roads? Roman war chariots formed the initial ruts, which everyone else had to match for fear of destroying their wagon wheels. Since the chariots were made for Imperial Rome, they were all alike in the matter of wheel spacing.

Therefore, the United States standard railroad gauge of 4 feet, 8.5 inches is derived from the original specifications for an Imperial Roman war chariot.

Bureaucracies live forever. So---the next time you are handed a Specification/Procedure/Process and wonder 'What horse's "behind" came up with it' you may be exactly right. Imperial Roman army chariots were made just wide enough to accommodate the rear ends of two war horses. (Two horses' behinds).

Now the twist to the story to validate what I first alluded to: When you see a Space Shuttle sitting on its launch pad, there are two big booster rockets attached to the sides of the main fuel tank. These are solid rocket boosters, or SRB's. The SRB's are made by Thiokol at their factory in Utah. The engineers who designed the SRB's would have preferred to make them a bit "fatter", but the SRB's had to be shipped by train from the factory to the launch site.

The railroad line from the factory happens to run through a tunnel in the mountains, and the SRB's had to fit through that tunnel. The tunnel is slightly wider than the railroad track, and the railroad track, as you now know, is about as wide as two horses behinds.

So---a major Space Shuttle design feature of what is arguably the world's most advanced transportation system was determined over two thousand years ago by the width of a horses behind. And you thought being a horses behind wasn't important. Ancient horse's ----- controlled almost everything and others are resisting change even today."

Now, to be sure, there are treatment agencies which have evolved into magnificent 21st century recovery centers. There are several around the country and to name just two there is Dr. Joan Larsons center and Colonial Clinic in WA state. But the majority of approaches dealing with patients, or clients, presenting for "treatment" do their best to 'talk the person into wellness'. They point out the damage done to the persons family, friends and co-workers. Shame will cause the addict to repent I suppose. They glowingly discuss "value systems" not really understanding that the 'client' has no idea what they are talking about. They spend hours discussing "family systems" and the effect that must have had on "causing the person to drink or drug". Over and over they insist the client attend a variety of classes and attempt to learn and retain information in a toxic brain. One effect of all this required and anticipated teaching and learning expectations is that the client is further convinced they are "less than" the rest of society. The client sees others as "having life in their hands and just living it". While the addicted person is suffering the ongoing relentless effects of withdrawal, with all of the varied negative symptoms, they are expected to begin making quality life decisions about what they will do in a society they judge as way above them intellectually and socially.

In other words, just as the man I interviewed at discharge from an inpatient treatment "experience" said - we take away their primary coping tools and leave them with all their problems.

As our experience with the "Railroad" has shown us, we just keep doing what we have always done because someone else did and it is easier than challenging the system. As I said earlier we used to present this information to Recovery Center directors in an effort to get them to see the need for change from their "railroad track" systems. Almost to a person they agreed it made sense but "did we have any idea how much training for counselors would be needed and how much time and effort it would take to change their operation manuals"? So, change never happened for most.

Information about family systems, about 'values clarification', about responsibility, and all the rest of varied classroom information can be important and meaningful IF it is presented at the correct time in recovery. A brain suffering the toxicity of alcohol or other drug use may take 6 months to just stabilize, and then only if the person is taking the correct steps to achieve this first stage of Maslow's hierarchy of needs.

It is time we started asking the clients to be involved in their own treatment planning, identifying with us their most pressing problems, guiding them in physiologic stabilization, recognizing when they can move to more problem solving, or determining what is preventing them from further progress, using education about addiction to alcohol, other drugs and dysfunctional behaviors when they are able to understand what is being talked about, actually doing individualized treatment, not "cookie cutter" or what ever is easier for the counselor or agency.

We could move to a very significant increase in the actual success in recovery if we are willing to learn and implement the skills needed to structure and guide recovery, not just focus on stopping the use of mind and mood altering chemicals or actions.

CHAPTER 22

Meeting the Maslow Defined Hierarchy Of Needs

Abraham Maslow is one of my heroes and he first introduced his concept of a hierarchy of needs in his 1943 paper "A Theory of Human Motivation" and his subsequent book, "Motivation and Personality". This "hierarchy" is most often displayed as a pyramid. The lowest levels of the pyramid are made up of the most basic needs, while the more complex needs are located at the top of the pyramid. Needs at the bottom of the pyramid (foundation of the pyramid) are the basic physical and physiological requirements for life. These include the need for healthy nutrition, water, sleep and warmth. Once these needs are being addressed, and only when the brain is aware they are being met, can a person then move on to the next level of needs, which are for safety and security. Safety and security needs include a desire for steady employment, safe neighborhoods, and shelter from the environment. Only if and when these needs are being addressed will the brain allow the person to use some daily energy to enter the next tier which involves socialization. Relationships such as friendships, romantic attachments and families help fulfill this need for companionship and acceptance. This is the time that AA or other 12 Step programs can be necessary and invaluable. Belonging to a "group" for support is best done only when the other needs have been addressed. After the first three levels of need have been satisfied the "esteem" needs become increasingly important. These include the need for things that reflect on self-esteem, personal growth, social recognition and accomplishment.

Only when these previous needs have been met can a person sense "self-actualization". People are then self-aware, concerned with personal growth, and interested in fulfilling their potential.

The progress attained in this quest can be explained and coordinated with the cessation of harmful chemical use and the insertion of quality nutrition and supplements to begin the repair of damaged neurochemical systems. A person is VERY UNLIKELY to achieve success in recovery without laying a solid foundation on which to build. Just as engineers know that any building must have an adequate and lasting foundation before they start to add floors to the project, so too must a person have a foundation in place before progressing toward being the best person they can become. Too often counselors want to start addressing "self-esteem" needs before the necessary foundations are in place and consequently the "building" falls down and the client is blamed as "just not being ready". The "client" is in front of you, the counselor, and it is your responsibility to understand how to correctly guide the recovery process and not attempt to "skip" steps crucial to positive development.

Remember the client interviewed as he was leaving an in-patient treatment experience? He knew he had to give up his primary coping tool, alcohol and drugs, but he still had no understanding how to address his physiological needs, his needs for safety and security, his needs for belonging and acceptance because he still had all of his life problems and no way to change them without proper guidance. Too often when we were attempting to move the treatment field toward the appropriate approaches for successful recovery did I hear "those things are not my job. My job is get him/

her to stop drinking and drugging". Stopping the use of mind and mood altering chemicals is not difficult. The difficult part is staying stopped. Short stays in an in-patient setting provide a safe place to detoxify and begin the very early process of brain recovery. This short stay is not capable, for most clients, of providing sufficient understandable information for ongoing recovery. Detoxification is necessary, and takes up to six months to complete.

Successful recovery from any addictive substance or maladaptive behavior is not easy. BUT, it is simple. Take the right steps in the right order!!

Structure and discipline. Just do it!

Summary of Suggestions for Supplement Use
1-800-862-5033
Physiological stabilization is vital to begin successful recovery. The following list provides the best starting program.

1. To overcome the effects of stress (trauma) use **NeuBecalmd.** Take 3 in the AM and 3 in afternoon. Try to take on empty stomach (if you forget take it anyway). DO NOT take at the same time as any medications being used.
2. To begin the stabilization from excessive alcohol use start with **Neu-Recover.** Take 3 in the morning and 3 in afternoon. Try to take on an empty stomach (but take it) and DO NOT take with other medications. After 90 days switch to **Neu-Becalmd** for ongoing repair and support.
3. To begin stabilization from any stimulant drug (ie cocaine, methamphetamine, or other arousal addictions such as gambling) use **Neu-Replenish.** Take 3 in morning and 3 in afternoon. Do NOT take at same time as other medications. After 90 days switch to NeuBecalmd for ongoing repair and support.
4. To begin stabilization in the withdrawal from prescription tranquilizer use (should be monitored by your physician)

use **Neu-Relieve.** Take 2 capsules 3 times a day. Do NOT take at the same time as you take the prescription tranquilizer. You MUST slowly, over time, very gradually reduce your tranquilizer use. A process as suggested by Heather Ashton for gradual withdrawal is a good guide. This may take several months to completely withdraw so patience is a must. Stay with **Neu-Relieve** throughout this process. When finally free from the medication, **NeuBecalmd** can be used for the ongoing support of stress management.

5. To assist in the withdrawal from opiate drugs (heroin, Demerol, codeine, methadone, etc) use a **Combination** of **Neu-Relieve and Neu-Becalmd.** Take 1 capsules of each 3 times over the day. Do NOT take at the same time as the opiate drug. Gradually reduce the opiate drug over time while taking the **Combo.**

For questions regarding other issues and for help with stabilization of other dependencies contact Neurogenesis at 1-800-862-5033 for referral.

www.ingramcontent.com/pod-product-compliance
Lightning Source LLC
Chambersburg PA
CBHW030346290526
45785CB00004B/1620